Quick & Easy Keto Cookbook for Beginners 2022

D1519095

BY: Batiste Velazquez

The Complete Guide of Ketogenic Diet weekly Meal Prepping Cookbook for Beginners and Advanced Users for Busy People on The Ketogenic Diet.

TABLE OF CONTENTS

INTRODUCTION

I have struggled with my weight almost for seemingly perpetually, since my teenager years. I've been on a tight eating routine since I was 14. I was reliably greedy; I didn't have a nice night's rest and energy for my consistently tasks and activities. Before long that, I slowed down in an example of "yo-yo counting calories" or weight gain followed by weight decrease. I went through various years feeling insane with my eating. I felt that I was disengaged from my own body and I didn't as yet focus on it I can't help myself. As a youth of 16, I fought with bitterness. I felt squashed; my partners couldn't understand how this straight-An understudy and beautiful youngster could have any mental issues. Besides, my people neglected to truly see what I was going through; they thought I went through a phase like various teens with fluctuating sentiments. A while later, when I was in school, my fights continued. I was eating less carbs, occasionally successfully sometimes not. It takes after a hamster on its wheel! Exactly when I graduated school, I had all that I thought I required. Taking everything into account, I was grieved. I had an essentially phobic nervousness toward food, especially slick food, nuts, and oily cheddar. This feeling about fats relies upon a regular reality that we have heard so frequently so we just expect it is legitimate. It takes after various contemplations that fall into the characterization of "legends" that are completely misguided! Amusingly, standard food, including ordinary fats, is truly extraordinary for the human body. On a fundamental level, to get fit, you ought to burn-through a greater number of calories than you eat; you should moreover zero in on standard proactive errands, utilize the flight of stairs instead of lifts, strolling an extra 30 minutes out of every day, blah, blah, blah... Easier said than done. Before long, we should inspect numerous factors to grasp that there is consistently more than one justification for weight gain. Mental factors, inherited tendency, food oppression, high insulin levels, synthetic disparity, and neurologic issues all may have an effect.

Exactly when I recollect my life, I see low certainty and terribleness. I furthermore accepted that cooking at home is monotonous so I reliably mentioned food transport. I decided to stop torturing myself and break the starve-gorge cycle. I decided to be content! "Everything in your life is an impression of a choice you have made. Accepting that you really want another result, make a substitute choice," said Anonymous. In any case, I asked myself, "What make you feel continually anxious, regardless of eating adequate food and three dinners each day? What are you doing to your body!? How might it be smart for you react to feel and put your best self forward?" These requests were tangled for me, yet some place down in my heart, I understood that the reactions were essential. Luckily, I found the reactions and retouch my relationship with food.

Three years earlier, I had found a low-carb dietary daily practice. It is a low starch, moderate protein, and high fat-based eating routine. Generally, I can eat meat, poultry, eggs and dairy on a keto diet and avoid rice, grains and vegetables. I was skeptical consistently, it sounds unreasonable! Fortunately, I was defamed; this food plan is better than I've anytime expected. My target with this recipe arrangement is to show you a basic yet strong way to deal with sendoff a ketogenic diet. Also, I expected to use my experience and data to help you on your keto experience with every single unpredictable detail. Following a really long time of fight, I feel confident and charged up to give preplanned grace and assist others with finding their direction to a merry life Assuming you feel overwhelmed or undermined, whatever you are going through, I am here to tell you that anything is possible; thusly, will not at any point give up. If I can do it, you can also!

WHAT IS THE KETO DIET?

As demonstrated by Wikipedia, "A ketogenic diet is an eating schedule that decides most of its calories from fat and only couple of calories from carbs. The eating routine powers the body to burn-through fats rather than carbs for energy. Regularly, the starches you eat are changed into glucose in the body, which is used for energy around the body and in the frontal cortex. Nonetheless, if you don't eat a satisfactory number of starches, your body has a back-up process for burning-through fat taking everything into account. The liver can use set aside fat and the fat you eat for energy. Set aside fat is broken into two areas, unsaturated fats, and ketone bodies. Ketone bodies power the brain rather than glucose. This state of having a huge load of ketone bodies in your blood is called Ketosis."

Exactly when I found a keto lifestyle, something about it really impelled me to do quick and dirty investigation. I read a huge load of articles and studies, seeing certifiable people getting authentic and mind-blowing results; then, I set up theory as an ordinary event and voilà! I did it! Likewise, I did it ably! A month right after starting this staggering lifestyle, my life completely changed.

I started after a ketogenic diet with a step-by-step calorie breakdown of 5% carbs, 20% protein, and 75% fats. I also endeavored to stay inside my calorie needs. It is simple since a run of the mill symptom of this eating routine is the vibe of fruition. The hankering camouflage may be associated with a higher affirmation of fat and protein. My conclusive goal was to help the body's processing to speed up my weight decrease. Other than being in ketosis, I endeavored to carry out specific enhancements to help fire up with expanding my processing. A piece of these movements fuse having a respectable breakfast, doing direct exercises to build muscles, having protein with every supper, drinking green tea, and adding hot peppers to my dinners. "Do whatever it takes not to skip dinners" is likely the best tip I've heard since skipping meals, especially breakfast, can make the absorption postponed down.

At the point when I showed up at my ideal weight, I endeavored to turn uncommonly low carb days with higher carb days so I can say that clear plan works for me. Then again, you can keep on with your keto lifestyle, but you can eat fairly greater sustenance for weight support. You can add fairly more protein yet keep carbs low. You can add more carbs just beforehand, then, at that point, afterward works out. It is fitting to go step by step, and raise your step-by-step carb limit by 10 to 20 grams for conceivably 14 days, and stick with Paleo food sources. In this stage, you can eat carbs that are supplement thick and fiber-rich like carrots, peppers, potatoes, turnips, pears, bananas, oranges, and strawberries. Another exceptional technique for staying aware of your true weight is to solidify unpredictable fasting with muscle-gaining keto. The key is just to find that ideal proportion of sustenance for your body, age and activity level.

By far most, including me, don't should be in ketosis to stay at a sound weight, as long as they stay with a low-carb diet, for instance, Paleo, LCHF or low-carb Mediterranean eating routine. Pretty much four years into keto, I am staying aware of my ideal weight, feeling freedom from food like the one I have never had.

Star Tip: Choose supplement stuffed food sources that can fulfill you more straightforward, and normally, you will eat less.

WHAT TO EAT ON A KETOGENIC DIET?

I made a positive keto-obliging food list so you can keep it in your shopping sack.

Vegetables: Lettuce (different sorts), greens (spinach, Swiss chard, collard, mustard greens, kale, and turnip); mushrooms, onion, garlic, asparagus, arugula, avocado, celery, squash, kohlrabi, book choy, radishes, broccoli tomatoes, cauliflower, zucchini, eggplant. With some restriction: artichokes, Brussels sprouts, broccoli, cauliflower, cucumbers, green beans, cabbage, okra, snap peas, snow peas, and fennel.

Natural items: Blackberries, cranberries, raspberries, lemon, lime, coconut, and tomatoes.

Meat and Poultry: Beef, pork, game, sheep, and veal, chicken, turkey and duck. Ground meat: Pork, cheeseburger, turkey, and mixed ground meat.

Lunch and Deli Meats: Bacon, pancetta, pepperoni, salami, suppressant, chorizo, ham, pastrami, prosciutto, and touch. With some restriction: bologna and mortadella.

Fish: Fatty fish, white fish, lobster, crab, shrimp, scallops, mussels, squid, shellfishes, and octopus.

Other keto-obliging food sources include: Herbs and flavors (new or dried); bouillon 3D squares and granules.

Sauces and Condiments: Mayonnaise, mustard, pureed tomatoes, vinegar, and hot sauce (try to check the sustenance real factors mark).

Canned food: fish anchovies, crab, salmon, sardines, tomato, sauerkraut, pickles, and olives (attempt to check the sustenance real factors mark).

Baking trimmings: almond flour, coconut flour, baking powder, baking pop, cocoa, vanilla concentrate, faint chocolate, and galactomannan powder.

Nut and Seed Butters: peanut butter, almond margarine, hazelnut spread, macadamia nut margarine, coconut spread, pecan spread, sunflower seed spread, walnut margarine, and tahini.

Vegetarian: Tempeh, tofu, full-fat coconut milk, jackfruit, healthy yeast, Shirataki noodles, Nori sheets, cooked sea development, Kelp noodles, Kelp chips.

Keto-Friendly Alcohol: Whiskey, alcohol, dries martini, vodka, and tequila. Sea development: Wakame, chlorella, nori, dulse, spirulina, and kelp.

Keto sugars: Stevia drops, Erythritol, and Monk fruit are zero carb sugars;

Splenda (sucralose-based sugar) has 0.5g of carbs per bundle (1 g); Erythritol has 4 grams of carbs per teaspoon (4 grams); Xylitol has 4 grams of carbs per teaspoon (4 grams);

FOOD ASSORTMENTS TO AVOID ON A KETOGENIC DIET

Grains and grain-like seeds: Rice, wheat, quinoa, oats, amaranth, grain, buckwheat, corn, millet Flours: Wheat flour, cornmeal, arrowroot, cornstarch, cassava, dal, and fava beans.

Starches: Starchy vegetables, soy, lentils, sago, custard, plantain, banana, and mesquite.

Sugars: All sorts of sugar and syrup (rice syrup, malt syrup, sorghum syrup, corn syrup, carob syrup, and high maltose corn syrup), grain malt, stick juice pearls, stick juice, cure, malt, rapider, muscovado, panocha, meager, agave nectar, molasses, honey, and maple syrup.

Taken care of vegetable oils and Trans fats: Diglycerides, shortening, vegetable shortening, margarine, unesterified oils, corn oil, cottonseed oil, grapeseed oil, safflower oil, and soybean oil.

Milk and lessened fat dairy things: scattered skim milk, low-fat yogurts, without fat spread substitutes, and diminished fat cheddar.

Modern office developed fish and eggs, took care of meat Fruits (other than berries) and dried natural items

Sugary refreshments: pop and energized drinks.

KETOGENIC KITCHEN MAKEOVER

To make your keto looking for food more straightforward, here is the overview of extra room basics on a keto diet. It will help you with saving money by not buying pointless things.

LOW-CARB FLOURS

1. Almond flour (1/4 cup or 28 grams of almond flour has around 160 calories and 6 grams of complete carbs);
2. Coconut flour (2 tablespoons or 18 grams of coconut flour has around 45 calories and 11 grams of outright carbs);
3. Flax feast (2 tablespoons or 14 grams of flax supper has very nearly 70 calories and 5 grams of hard and fast carbs);
4. Sunflower seed dinner and Pumpkin seed supper.

SWEETENER: Stevia, Xylitol, Erythritol.

- NUTS and SEEDS
- CREAM CHEESE
- COCONUT MILK and COCONUT CREAM
- COCONUT OIL, AVOCADO OIL and OLIVE OIL
- MEAT, POULTRY and SEAFOOD
- NUT BUTTERS
- KETO VEGETABLES and FROZEN VEGETABLES

CONDIMENTS: Mustard, mayonnaise, Sirach, hot sauce, and vinegar.

- CACAO POWDER, CACAO NIBS and SUGAR-FREE DARK
- CHOCOLATE
- PSYLLIUM HUSKS

HERBS & SPICES: pink salt, sage, thyme, rosemary, dull pepper, oregano, basil, ginger, turmeric, and cinnamon.

MACRONUTRIENT BALANCE

Macronutrients ("macros") fuse protein, fat, and carbs. Macronutrients give energy as calories. For instance, fat gives 9 calories for every gram; then, there are 4 calories for each gram of protein; concerning carbs, there are 4 calories for each gram. Luckily, you can work out your keto macros quickly by using the Keto Calculator on the web. It can help you with finding the particular proportion of macronutrients you truly need to show up at your level headed, whether or not you really want to lose or stay aware of your weight. There are little PCs for a model ketogenic diet (75% fat, 20% protein, 5% sugar) and various assortments of keto thins down so you can incorporate unequivocal proportions of macros as shown by your tendency.

FATS (LIPIDS) are a key piece of a ketogenic diet. The sort of fats you eat on a keto diet is major since specific fats are better for weight decrease and more grounded than others. It took me long to understand that I need to eat fat to consume fat. Accepting you avoid fat and eat a ton of lean protein food assortments, for instance, skinless chicken and fish, the excess protein will be changed over into glucose. It can raise your insulin levels, also. Low-fat things may have all the earmarks of being a good decision for weight decrease since fats have been given a horrible standing already. In any case, reduced fat peanut butter, without fat serving of leafy greens dressings or low-fat yogurt regularly contain a huge load of sad trimmings, took care of oil, and sugar. The trick here is to eat more fat. For example, I should add spread to my morning feast, it finishes me off and helps me with having less at lunch. Recall that the human body needs a wide scope of fats including unsaturated fats and drenched fats. There are two essential sorts of unsaturated fats: 1) polyunsaturated fats (consolidate omega-3 fats and omega-6 fats), and 2) monounsaturated fats. Wellsprings of monounsaturated unsaturated fats fuse olive oil, nut oil, canola oil, sesame oil, and cashews. Food sources with a higher proportion of polyunsaturated fat fuse nuts, seeds, soybean oil, and oily fish. Food sources with higher proportions of splashed fats join oily cheeseburger, margarine, cheddar, pork, poultry with skin, cream, and fat. There is another class called "Trans fats" that are unsaturated fats that have been taken care of. You should eat less drenched and trans-fats to cut down the risk of coronary ailment, high blood cholesterol, and weight. To outline, inferior quality sustenance and packaged food sources contain absorbed fat a greater total. As such, you should avoid snack food hotspots, (for instance, oily potato chips), seared food sources, high fat significant point food sources (counting pizza, pasta, burgers), high-fat cakes, rolls, and rolls, cakes (like pies and croissants). Truly take a gander at the names and pick the things that are higher in poly and monounsaturated fats and lower in drenched and trans-fats. Remember, it is fundamental to eat fats in restricted amounts as a piece of a sensible ketogenic diet.

PROTEIN in like manner expects an outstanding part in the human body. It contains more humble units called amino acids; you need basic amino acids for your body to work properly. The fundamental components of proteins fuse the arrangement of synthetic substances, keeping a sound weight, propelling life expectancy, muscle improvement and fix. Protein is fundamental for a skin, bone, and psyche prosperity, also. Animal protein sources on a keto diet join fish, meat, poultry, cheddar, and eggs. Plant protein sources consolidate commonly nuts and seeds.

There are different viewpoints on protein utilization on a keto diet. Some ketogenic experts propose high protein affirmation (1 gram of protein for each 1 pound). A couple of experts advocates low protein affirmation for people who follow a keto diet or 1.0 grams of protein per kilogram of lean mass (2.2 pounds). They acknowledge excess protein can change into sugar in your body and thwart ketosis. There is the third assembling of experts that proposes 1.5-1.75 grams of protein per 2.2 pounds. By far most agree that we should follow this formula to enter and stay in ketosis 5% carbs, 20% protein, and 75% fats. Sugars are macronutrients that the human body converts to glucose; to be sure, glucose is the body's main fuel source. Your organs like kidneys, frontal cortex, and heart all need carbs to work fittingly. Moreover, fats can't be true to form used without carbs as fiber that is needed for ingestion. Other than being a fuel, glucose can be taken care of as glycogen in our liver or muscles. Put forward evidently, overconsumption of carbs extends the development of fatter storing. The human body moreover requires micronutrients, including supplements and minerals. Recollect that the vast majority of micronutrients and critical phytonutrients come from vegetables; it infers that you should eat a gigantic piece of keto veggies with each gala. Right when you know your macros, you can without a very remarkable stretch game plan your day on a ketogenic diet.

6 CRITICAL KETOGENIC DIET TIPS

You should make time to start your day right. Throwing a fair breakfast with protein and sound fats, for instance, an omelet or egg rolls, will control your eating throughout the day. Eating a sound low-carb breakfast can basically restore the glucose levels in your body a lot of like your vehicle needs fuel to run. You should focus in on having protein-rich food sources like milk, nuts, seeds, and eggs. Skipping breakfast impacts demeanor and intellectual ability. Similarly, it may incite hypertension, raised cholesterol, and hypertension. Investigates have shown that people who skip breakfast have obvious levels of fatigue throughout the span of the day.

Expecting you think you miss the mark on ability to manage breakfast, this equation collection may help you with beating that issue. This variety expresses straightforward breakfast impressions like egg bread rolls, keto fat bombs, low-carb pancakes; and so, on You can in like manner change dinner additional items into a go-to breakfast. A dish with eggs and bacon that is done off with sharp cheddar makes an extraordinary unwinding dinner similarly as an in and out breakfast. Make-ahead breakfast is brilliant idea for those in a hurry, too. For instance, you can make lettuce wraps, chicken plate of leafy greens or cheddar crisps and store them in invulnerable holders up to 3 days. You can make a cheddar and vegetable gratin in Sunday morning; it will in general be warmed quickly or liked cold straightforwardly from the refrigerator. With our keto plans, you can without a very remarkable stretch make feast prep a penchant! Remember, your body needs to refuel first thing. Thus, take your morning dinner inside an hour of enlivening. Breakfast is a spectacularly critical key to a productive keto diet and to better prosperity.

SORT OUT SOME WAY TO USE THE FOOD REAL FACTORS MARK.

Most importantly, keep carbs low. It will help you with making better food choices that add to your eating routine. Then, check for covered sugars, which is "enemy number one" on a keto diet. Most dealt with food assortments contain stowed away sugar since it overhauls flavor and helps defend food sources. Ordinary sugars join rough sugar, hearty hued sugar, sucrose, sugar syrup, high-fructose corn syrup, switch sugar, normal sugar, corn syrup, Turbinado, corn sugar, dextrose, fructose, natural item squeeze consolidated, maltose, glucose, lactose, malt syrup, and Sorghum syrup. They don't contribute any clinical benefits to your dinners.

You should moreover avoid the going with trimmings: caramel, stick juice, stick juice solids, dextrin, dextran, grain malt, beet sugar, buttered syrup, carob syrup, date sugar, diastase, diastatic malt, splendid syrup, Refiner's syrup, and ethyl maltol.

Experiences have shown that the typical American consumes something like 64 pounds of sugar every year or 22 teaspoons of added sugars a day. Concerning sound keto sugars, you should choose a sugar that is made of ordinary trimmings and doesn't contain engineered substances. Besides, you should pick a sugar that has dietary advantage yet you'll regardless be inside your step-by-step carb limit. Stevia and minister natural item are typical sugars that give clinical benefits. Stevia is on different occasions better compared to sugar and no influences glucose levels. When purchasing stevia, look for a pure, regular thing. Cleric normal item is a zero-calorie sugar; studies have exhibited that minister regular item has basic quieting and malignant growth counteraction specialist properties. It is useful in diminishing exacerbation and controlling insulin flexibility.

SORT OUT SOME WAY TO GATHER MUSCLE ON A KETO DIET.

Building thin mass is critical for a powerful ketogenic diet since you will consume off your muscle versus fat's stores even more capably. There are four sorts of exercises I achieved for assisting muscle with measuring: Deadlifts, up press, squats, and seat press.

It's essential to refuel your body with supplement thick keto sustenance for ideal athletic execution. In addition, give close thought to your electrolyte usage. For example, low-carb, potassium-rich food assortments fuse mushrooms, spinach, broccoli, and salmon. Low-carb, magnesium-rich food assortments fuse almonds, avocados, and faint chocolate. The body similarly loses sodium, chloride, and calcium during exercise.

FIND OUT NET CARBS.

I understand it might be puzzling to figure out how much carbs to join into your step-by-step feast plan. Sorting out some way to discover net carbs is essential for progress on a keto diet. Without a doubt, net carbs are the starches that our body can process and uses for energy. Hold fast to the formula: Total Carbohydrate - Dietary Fiber - Sugar Alcohol = Net Carbs. Dietary fiber and sugar alcohol (most of them) are non-consumable carbs. Your liver doesn't use non-absorbable carbs to change over them into glucose. Likewise, net carbs simply count starches and sugars.

By the day's end, you don't need to join sugar alcohols (xylitol, mannitol, lactitol, and erythritol) into your carb limit assessments. On the other hand, each gram of sorbitol, is malt, maltitol, or glycerin considers around 0.5 gram of carbs. Further, fiber is totally recorded under carbs anyway our body can't manage them; they don't have an energy a motivating force for the human body. They are generally recorded under "Dietary Fiber" on food names. Dissolvable dietary fiber accepts an indispensable part in the rule of desiring by achieving settled insulin levels. Further, the method for sounding low-carb excluding calories is to find about macronutrients and what they mean for your body. Appropriately, you should consider working out your net carbs as opposed to amounting to carbs. Accepting you are a beginner, pay special attention to covered carbs.

PONDER ENERGY THICKNESS.

To be sure, energy thickness is the number of calories per gram of food. Regarding a keto diet, it is reasonable to base you're eating routine course of action around medium energy thickness food sources and eat higher energy thickness food assortments in unobtrusive amounts. Of course, lower energy thickness food assortments have fewer calories per gram of food. They join clear soups and stews similarly as vegetables and fundamental nursery plates of leafy greens that are typically high in water.

EAT CERTIFIED FOOD.

This suggests that on a ketogenic diet you'll need to eat whole, normal food that is rich in supplements. It is basic to avoid engineered added substances and terrible sustenance. Focusing in on whole, regular and grass-dealt with food assortments will make your life more direct and your body better.

3 PROVEN BENEFITS OF A KETOGENIC DIET

1. A keto diet prompts weight decrease. Exactly when you avoid sugars, your body starts consuming set aside fat; it will thus cause lessened needing. Of course, you will experience higher energy levels.

2. Mental clarity and better obsession. On a keto diet, our frontal cortex includes ketones as the basic fuel; along these lines, it lessens the levels of toxins. It will through and through additionally foster your intellectual abilities, mental focus, obsession, and mental execution.

3. Health benefits. A keto diet limits starches; they can be found in bothersome sweet food assortments, refined grains like bread, pasta and white rice. Of course, it propels food assortments that are stacked with incredible protein (it is central for building muscle), extraordinary fat, and strong veggies. Numerous assessments have shown that low-carb diets can generally additionally foster prosperity. They assessed the essential outcomes, for instance, LDL cholesterol, HDL cholesterol, glucose levels, greasy substances, and weight decrease.
Oily fish such (for example, fish and salmon) is remarkable for its ability to cut down greasy substances; thusly, it can lessen the risk of stroke. Unsaturated fat-squeezed food assortments, for instance, seeds, nuts and rough vegetable oils can help your body with cutting down greasy oils, also. Likewise, eliminating carbs can decrease insulin levels and control glucose. Not solely can keto consume less calories further foster your real execution and lift weight decrease, but they moreover treat a couple of significant conditions. Keto thins down have exhibited supportive in dealing with a couple of brain issues like epilepsy in youths. Moreover, ketogenic eats less are incomprehensibly effective in treating metabolic confusion.

A FEW HACKS YOU MIGHT BENEFIT FROM

Stay hydrated: According to the United States National Library of Medicine, an adult individual should drink between 2.7 to 3.7 liters of water every day. Be mindful with regards to liquid calories on a ketogenic diet. Avoid alcohol and further developed refreshments; you can satisfy your thirst with gleaming water (with added new lemon juice), full-fat yogurt, or ice tea. Eat new vegetables that are regularly high in water content. As various keto-errs, I experienced dry mouth and awful breath, also; they are ordinary signs of ketosis. How I discard ketosis breath? Attempt to brush reliably, chomp sans sugar gum, and drink more water.

Fat coffee: This is my personal business to consuming fat speedier. A few coffees with a tablespoon of spread give me a somewhat long energy hit until early afternoon. I love its perfection and especially waiting flavor and I am astonished by its results. It may sound crazy, yet endeavor it once and you will go completely gaga for "fat dim".

Keep it essential: The way in to a viable ketogenic diet is working on changes to your lifestyle. Make a direct ketogenic feast expect to end up stirred up with a regular practice; stick to basic plans like servings of leafy greens and soups. Go for essential goodies, also. Tidy up and enhance your kitchen, and pick quick dinners to get ready at home.

Surrender control, loosen up and head outside. Getting outside air and contributing energy with family or pets will help with making you bound to hold fast to your eating schedule.

21-DAY MEAL PLAN

I made an easy to-follow dinner plan for you to send off your keto adventure right. This is a model menu for a seriously lengthy timespan on a ketogenic diet plan.

DAY 1

Breakfast: 1 tablespoon of peanut butter; 1 cut of keto bread

Lunch: Easy Turkey Curry; 1 unassuming pack of ice sheet lettuce

Dinner: Smoked Haddock Fish Burgers; 1 medium tomato

DAY 2

Breakfast: 1 hard-percolated egg; 1 cut of bacon; 1 shake with 1/2 cup of coconut milk and protein powder

Lunch: Classic Beef Stroganoff; 1 serving of cauliflower rice

Dinner: Alaskan Cod with Mustard Cream Sauce; 1 medium tomato

DAY 3

Breakfast: Paprika Omelet with Goat Cheese; 5-6 almonds

Lunch: Chinese Ground Beef Skillet; 1 cup rough kid spinach with squeezed apple vinegar

Dinner: Special Chicken Salad; 1 keto dinner roll

DAY 4

Breakfast: Omelet with veggies; 1 cut of bacon

Lunch: Pork Cutlets in Chili Tangy Sauce; 1 serving of coleslaw

Dinner: Lemon Garlic Grilled Chicken Wings; 1 medium tomato

DAY 5

Breakfast: Dilly Boiled Eggs with Avocado; a touch of bitter cream; 1-2 pickles

Lunch: Beef Shredded Beef with Herbs; 1 unassuming bundle of mixed green plate of leafy greens in with a few showers of a recently squeezed lemon juice

Dinner: Two-Cheese Zucchini Gratin; 1 teaspoon of mustard

DAY 6

Breakfast: Greek-Style Frittata with Herbs; 1 keto roll

Lunch: Holiday Pork Belly with Vegetables; 1 serving of cauliflower rice

Dinner: Ranch and Blue Cheese Dip; Greek-style salad (tomato, cucumber, ringer peppers, feta cheddar)

DAY 7

Breakfast: Mangalorean Egg Curry

Lunch: Italian Zuppa di Pomodoro; 1 gigantic tomato; 1 cup of seared mushrooms with 1 tablespoon of margarine

Dinner: Ranch Chicken Wings; Cheese and Artichoke Dip

DAY 8

Breakfast: Scrambled eggs; 1 tomato; 1/2 cup of Greek-style yogurt

Lunch: Cheeseburger Skillet with Bacon and Mushrooms; 1 serving of cauliflower rice

Dinner: Swedish Herring Salad

DAY 9

Breakfast: Egg, Bacon and Kale Muffins; 1/2 cup unsweetened almond milk

Lunch: Hearty Fisherman's Stew; 1 serving of cabbage salad

Dinner: Two-Cheese and Kale Bake

DAY 10

Breakfast: Cauliflower, Cheese and Egg Fat Bombs

Lunch: Grandma's Zucchini and Spinach Chowder; 1/2 chicken chest; 1 scallion

Dinner: Italian Cheddar Crisps; a hint of bitter cream; 2 tablespoons tomato stick

DAY 11

Breakfast: 1 tablespoon of peanut butter; 1 cut of keto bread

Lunch: Country-Style Pork Stew; 1 serving of cabbage salad

Dinner: Cauliflower, Ham and Cheese Bake

DAY 12

Breakfast: The Best Zucchini Fritters Ever; 1/2 cup of full-fat Greek yogurt

Lunch: Filipino Nilaja Soup; 1 serving of low-carb grilled vegetables

Dinner: Peanut Butter Cubes

DAY 13

Breakfast: Crêpes with Peanut Butter and Coconut

Lunch: Creamy Broccoli and Bacon Soup; 1 medium cucumber; 1 stewed chicken drumstick

Dinner: Mexican-Style Pork Tacos

DAY 14

Breakfast: Vanilla Mug Cake

Lunch: Cheesy Zucchini Casserole; 1 humble pack of kid spinach with 1 teaspoon of mustard and 1 teaspoon of olive oil

Dinner: Turkey Crust Pizza with Bacon

DAY 15

Breakfast: Easiest Brownies Ever

Lunch: Salmon Curry with a Twist; 1 serving of stewed keto veggies

Dinner: Stuffed Spaghetti Squash Bowls

DAY 16

Breakfast: Deviled Eggs with Mustard and Chives; 1/2 cup of Greek-style yogurt

Lunch: Ranch Chicken Breasts with Cheese

Dinner: Spicy Baked Eggplant with Herbs and Cheese; Almond Butter and Chocolate Cookies

DAY 17

Breakfast: 2 hard-percolated eggs; 2 cuts of cheddar

Lunch: Pork Tenderloin with Southern Cabbage; 1 cut of keto bread

Dinner: Italian-Style Spicy Meatballs; 1 cucumber

DAY 18

Breakfast: Lettuce Wraps with Ham and Cheese

Lunch: Stuffed Peppers with Cauliflower and Cheese; 1/2 grilled chicken chest

Dinner: Smoked Haddock Fish Burgers

DAY 19

Breakfast: Double Cheese and Sausage Balls

Lunch: Indian-Style Fried Pork; 1 serving of steamed broccoli; 1 cucumber

Dinner: 1 grilled pork sausage; 1 teaspoon Dijon mustard; Chinese-Style Cauliflower Rice

DAY 20

Breakfast: Cheesy Brussels sprouts; 1 medium tomato with 2-3 Kalamata olives

Lunch: Spinach with Paprika and Cheese; 1 hint of sharp cream

Dinner: Rich Double-Cheese Meatloaf

DAY 21

Breakfast: Mini Stuffed Peppers; 1 serving of blue cheddar

Lunch: Holiday Pork Belly with Vegetables; 1 serving of cabbage salad

Dinner: 1 steamed chicken chest; 1 serving of stewed asparagus; Peanut Butter and Chocolate Treat If you get enthusiastic between meals, there are strong, keto goodies that can finish you off. They consolidate a few hard-gurgled eggs, kid carrots with tablespoon or two of a keto plunging sauce, full-fat yogurt with tablespoon or two of new berries, a little bundle of nuts, and a few cheddar sticks.

CONCERNING OUR RECIPE COLLECTION

My goal with this book is to help and animate people who decide to carry out a positive improvement in their lives. Along these lines, this book features 75 plans, from essential designs for new keto-errs to cheerful plans that everyone will love, so you never run out of considerations.

These plans are made with ordinary trimmings that pass on mind blowing flavor and astonishing scents. They are upheld by my significant other and my guests who consistently come over for dinner. They are expected to guide you continually to set up the best keto food wellsprings ever. Each equation consolidates the sustaining information and has as much as 6 grams of net carbs. These are the best method for following your macronutrients and adjust your eating routine to oblige your noteworthy necessities. Other than being an inconceivable focal point for keto plans, the book is packed with cooking special experiences, insightful tricks, and accommodating hacks. Might it be said that you are good to go keto? Continue! Remember, expecting I can get it going, you can also!

VEGETABLES and SIDE DISHES

1. CAULIFLOWER, HAM AND CHEESE BAKE

Prepared in around: 40 minutes

Servings: 4

This smooth feast tastes so magnificent! Cauliflower joins magnificently with ham, cheddar, Greek-yogurt and Mediterranean flavors.

Per serving:

- 188 Calories;
- 11.3g Fat;
- 5.7g Carbs;
- 1.1g Fiber;
- 14.9g Protein;
- 2.9g Sugars

Fixings:

- 1/2 teaspoon butter, melted
- 1 (1/2-pound) head cauliflower, broken into florets
- 1/2 cup Swiss cheese, shredded
- 1/2 cup Mexican blend cheese, room temperature
- 1/2 cup Greek-style yogurt
- 1 cup cooked ham, chopped
- 1 roasted chili pepper, chopped
- 1/2 teaspoon porcini powder
- 1 teaspoon garlic powder
- 1 teaspoon shallot powder
- 1/2 teaspoon cayenne pepper
- 1/4 teaspoon dried sage
- 1/2 teaspoon dried Oregano Sea
- Salt and ground black pepper, to taste

Headings

Start by preheating your grill to 340 degrees F. Then, coat the base and sides of a goulash dish with 1/2 teaspoon of melted spread.

Void the cauliflower into a pot and cover it with water. Permit it to cook for 6 minutes until it is very fragile (mash able). Squash the coordinated cauliflower with a potato ricer press or potato masher.

As of now, blend in the cheddar; blend until the cheddar has relaxed. Add Greek-style yogurt, cut ham, cooked pepper, and flavors.

Place the mix in the set-up goulash dish; plan in the preheated oven for 20 minutes. Permit it to sit for around 10 minutes before cutting. Serve and appreciate!

2. RICH BROCCOLI AND BACON SOUP

Prepared in around: 20 minutes

Servings: 4

This rich soup will help you with keeping your eating routine on track. It might be refrigerated up to 3 days.

Per serving:

- 95 Calories;
- 7.6g Fat;
- 4.1g Carbs;
- 1g Fiber;
- 3g Protein;
- 1.7g Sugars

Fixings:

- 2 slices bacon, chopped
- 2 tablespoons scallions, chopped
- 1 carrot, chopped
- 1 celery, chopped Salt and ground black pepper, to taste
- 1 teaspoon garlic, finely chopped
- 1/2 teaspoon dried rosemary
- 1 sprig thyme, stripped and chopped
- 1/2 head green cabbage, shredded
- 1/2 head broccoli, broken into small florets
- 3 cups water
- 1 cup chicken stock
- 1/2 cup full-fat yogurt

Headings

Heat a stockpot over medium hotness; as of now, consume the bacon until new. Hold the bacon and 1 tablespoon of fat.

Then, cook scallions, carrots, and celery in 1 tablespoon of held fat. Add salt, pepper, and garlic; cook an additional 1 second or until fragrant.

By and by, blend in rosemary, thyme, cabbage, and broccoli. Pour in water and stock, bringing to a quick air pocket; reduce hotness and let it stew for 10 minutes more.

Add yogurt and cook an additional 5 minutes, mixing sometimes. Use a submersion blender, to puree your soup until smooth.

Taste and change the flavors. Adorn with the cooked bacon not long before serving.

3.SPINACH WITH PAPRIKA AND CHEESE

Prepared in around: 10 minutes

Servings: 4

Make a popular side dish in a brief time frame and daze your guests! Other typical additions to this recipe join Parmesan cheddar, nutmeg and flavors.

Per serving:

- 166 Calories;
- 15.1g Fat;
- 5g Carbs;
- 1.7g Fiber;
- 4.4g Protein;
- 2.1g Sugars

Fixings:

- 1 tablespoon butter, room temperature
- 1 clove garlic, minced
- 10 ounces spinach
- 1/2 teaspoon garlic salt
- 1/4 teaspoon ground black pepper or more to taste
- 1/2 teaspoon cayenne pepper
- 3 ounces cream cheese
- 1/2 cup double cream

Headings

Melt the spread in a pot that is preheated over medium hotness. Once hot. Cook garlic for 30 seconds.

As of now, add the spinach; cover the quest for gold minutes to permit the spinach to shrivel. Season with salt, dim pepper, and cayenne pepper Stir in cheddar and cream; blend until the cheddar breaks down. Serve immediately.

4.MUDDLED ZUCCHINI CASSEROLE

Prepared in around: 50 minutes

Servings: 4

This is a remarkable technique for spending the overflow of zucchini all through the mid-year season. You will worship this basic cheddar goulash!

Per serving:

- 155 Calories;
- 12.9g Fat;
- 3.5g Carbs;
- 0.8g Fiber;
- 7.6g Protein;
- 0.2g Sugars

Fixings:

- Nonstick cooking spray
- 2 cups zucchini, thinly sliced
- 2 tablespoons leeks, sliced
- 1/2 teaspoon salt Freshly ground black pepper, to taste
- 1/2 teaspoon dried basil
- 1/2 teaspoon dried oregano
- 1/2 cup Cheddar cheese, grated
- 1/4 cup heavy cream
- 4 tablespoons Parmesan cheese, freshly grated
- 1 tablespoon butter, room temperature
- 1 teaspoon fresh garlic, minced

Headings

Start by preheating your grill to 370 degrees F. Delicately oil a goulash dish with a nonstick cooking sprinkle.

Place 1 cup of the zucchini cuts in the dish; add 1 tablespoon of leeks; sprinkle with salt, pepper, basil, and oregano. Top with 1/4 cup of cheddar. Reiterate the layers indeed.

In a mixing dish, totally whisk the profound cream with Parmesan, margarine, and garlic. Spread this mix over the zucchini layer and cheddar layers.

Place in the preheated oven and hotness for around 40 to 45 minutes until the edges are well sautéed. Sprinkle with hacked chives, at whatever point needed. Bon appétit.

5. STUFFED PEPPERS WITH CAULIFLOWER AND CHEESE

Prepared in around: 45 minutes

Servings: 6

Over the ground vegetables, for instance, ringer pepper and cauliflower are overall extraordinary keto decisions while underground vegetables contain more carbs. These peppers are delicious served hot or cold. Appreciate!

Per serving:

- 244 Calories;
- 12.9g Fat;
- 3.2g Carbs;
- 1g Fiber;
- 16.5g Protein;
- 1.6g Sugars

Fixings:

- 2 tablespoons vegetable oil
- 2 tablespoons yellow onion, chopped
- 1 teaspoon fresh garlic, crushed
- 1/2-pound ground pork
- 1/2-pound ground turkey
- 1 cup cauliflower rice
- 1/2 teaspoon sea salt
- 1/4 teaspoon red pepper flakes, crushed
- 1/2 teaspoon ground black pepper
- 1 teaspoon dried parsley flakes
- 6 medium-sized bell peppers, deveined and cleaned
- 1/2 cup tomato sauce
- 1/2 cup Cheddar cheese, shredded

Headings

Heat the oil in a skillet over medium fire. Once hot, sauté the onion and garlic for 2 to 3 minutes.

Add the ground meat and cook for 6 minutes longer or until it is well caramelized. Add cauliflower rice and planning. Continue to cook for a further 3 minutes.

Split the filling between the set-up ringer peppers. Cover with a piece of foil.

Place the peppers in a baking holder; add pureed tomatoes.

Heat in the preheated oven at 380 degrees F for 20 minutes. Uncover, top with cheddar, and plan for 10 minutes more. Bon appétit!

6.CHINESE-STYLE CAULIFLOWER RICE

Prepared in around: 15 minutes

Servings: 3

This Asian-style omelet with cauliflower is overflowing with sound keto food assortments. You can add some bean stew for an extra kick, at whatever point needed.

Per serving:

- 131 Calories;
- 8.9g Fat;
- 6.2g Carbs;
- 1.8g Fiber;
- 7.2g Protein;
- 2.2g Sugars

Fixings:

- 1/2-pound fresh cauliflower
- 1 tablespoon sesame oil
- 1/2 cup leeks, chopped
- 1 garlic pressed Sea salt and freshly ground black pepper, to taste
- 1/2 teaspoon Chinese five-spice powder
- 1 teaspoon oyster sauce
- 1/2 teaspoon light soy sauce
- 1 tablespoon Shaoxing wine
- 3 eggs

Headings

Beat the cauliflower in a food processor until it seems as though rice.

Heat the sesame oil in a skillet over medium-high hotness; sauté the leeks and garlic for 2 to 3 minutes. Add the coordinated cauliflower rice to the skillet, close by salt, dull pepper, and Chinese five-flavor powder.

Then, at that point, add shellfish sauce, soy sauce, and wine. Permit it to cook, mixing occasionally, until the cauliflower is new fragile, around 5 minutes.

Then, add the eggs to the skillet; blend until everything is generally united.

Serve warm and appreciate!

7.LIVELY BAKED EGGPLANT WITH HERBS AND CHEESE

Prepared in around: 2 hours 45 minutes

Servings: 6

Eggplant is warmed between layers of Italian cheddar, kale, and garlic-tomato pasta sauce, making this Italian-breathed life into supper exceptionally scrumptious! You can add several sprinkles of other Italian flavors like parsley and sage, at whatever point needed. You can in like manner adorn your dish with new flavors for an extra flavor and shockingly better show.

Per serving:

- 230 Calories;
- 18.5g Fat;
- 6.7g Carbs;
- 2.4g Fiber;
- 10.6g Protein;
- 3.3g Sugars

Fixings:

- 1 (3/4-pound) eggplant, cut into
- 1/2-inch slices
- 1 tablespoon olive oil
- 1 tablespoon butter, melted
- 8 ounces kale leaves, torn into pieces
- 14 ounces garlic- and-tomato pasta sauce, without sugar
- 1/3 cup cream cheese
- 1 cup Asiago cheese, shredded
- 1/2 cup Gorgonzola cheese, grated
- 3 tablespoons ketchup, without sugar
- 1 teaspoon Pepperoncino (hot pepper)
- 1 teaspoon Basilica (basil)
- 1 teaspoon oregano
- 1/2 teaspoon Rosmarinus (rosemary)

Headings

Place the eggplant cuts in a colander and sprinkle them with salt. License it to sit for 2 hours. Wipe the eggplant cuts with paper towels.

Brush the eggplant cuts with olive oil; cook in a cast-iron grill compartment until well sautéed on the different sides, around 5 minutes.

Condense the margarine in a dish over medium fire. By and by, cook the kale leaves until shriveled. In a mixing bowl, join the three sorts of cheddar.

Move the grilled eggplant slices to a tenderly lubed baking dish. Top with the kale. Then, add a layer of 1/2 of cheddar blend.

Pour the pureed tomatoes over the cheddar layer. Top with the overabundance cheddar mix. Sprinkle with getting ready.

Get ready in the preheated oven at 350 degrees F until cheddar is murmuring and splendid brown, around 35 minutes. Bon appétit!

8. THE BEST ZUCCHINI FRITTERS EVER

Prepared in around: 40 minutes

Servings: 6

These squanders are fast and easy to plan for dinner. Present with a touch of sharp cream, at whatever point needed. You can serve them as a side, also.

Per serving:

- 111 Calories;
- 8.9g Fat;
- 3.2g Carbs;
- 1g Fiber;
- 5.8g Protein;
- 0.5g Sugars.

Fixings:

- 1 pound zucchini, grated and drained
- 1 egg
- 1 teaspoon fresh Italian parsley
- 1/2 cup almond meal
- 1/2 cup goat cheese, crumbled Sea salt and ground black pepper, to taste
- 1/2 teaspoon red pepper flakes, crushed
- 2 tablespoons olive oil

Headings

Mix all trimmings, beside the olive oil, in a gigantic bowl. Permit it to sit in your cooler for 30 minutes.

Heat the oil into a non-stick frying pan over medium hotness; scoop the heaped tablespoons of the zucchini mix into the hot oil.

Cook for 3 to 4 minutes; then, gently flip the wastes over and cook on the contrary side. Cook in a couple of clusters.

Move to a paper towel to ingest any overflow oil. Serve and appreciate!

9.STUFFED SPAGHETTI SQUASH BOWLS

Prepared in around: 1 hour

Servings: 4

All of the sorts of your treasured pasta are full into these consumable dishes, but they are keto-obliging and faultless! These dishes look genuinely luxurious, they are sensible for any occasion.

Per serving:

- 219 Calories;
- 17.5g Fat;
- 6.9g Carbs;
- 0.9g Fiber;
- 9g Protein; 4.1g Sugars

Fixings:

- 1/2-pound spaghetti squash, halved, scoop out seeds
- 1 teaspoon olive oil
- 1/2 cup Mozzarella cheese, shredded
- 1/2 cup cream cheese
- 1/2 cup full-fat Greek yogurt
- 2 eggs
- 1 garlic clove, minced
- 1/2 teaspoon cumin
- 1/2 teaspoon basil
- 1/2 teaspoon mint Sea salt and ground black pepper, to taste

Headings

Place the squash parts in a baking compartment; sprinkle the inner pieces of each squash half with olive oil.

Heat in the preheated grill at 370 degrees F for 45 to 50 minutes or until the inner parts are easily penetrated through with a fork Now, fix the spaghetti squash "noodles" from the skin in a mixing bowl. Add the abundance trimmings and mix to join well. Circumspectly fill all of the squash half with the cheddar mix. Plan at 350 degrees F for 5 to 10 minutes, until the cheddar is permeating and splendid brown. Bon appétit!

POULTRY

10. TART CLASSIC CHICKEN DRUMETTES

Prepared in around: 40 minutes

Servings: 4

A ketogenic dinner shouldn't be tangled. Direct trimmings chicken, lemon, garlic. Irrelevant work-most prominent outcome!

Per serving:

- 209 Calories;
- 12.2g Fat;
- 0.4g Carbs;
- 0.1g Fiber;
- 23.2g Protein;
- 0.1g Sugars

Fixings:

- 1 pound chicken drumettes
- 1 tablespoon olive oil
- 2 tablespoons butter, melted
- 1 garlic clove, sliced Fresh juice of 1/2 lemon
- 2 tablespoons white wine Salt and ground black pepper, to taste
- 1 tablespoon fresh scallions, chopped

Headings

Start by preheating your grill to 440 degrees F. Place the chicken in a material lined baking skillet. Sprinkle with olive oil and melted margarine. Add the garlic, lemon, wine, salt, and dull pepper.

Get ready in the preheated oven for around 35 minutes. Serve adorned with new scallions. Appreciate!

11.BASIC TURKEY CURRY

Prepared in around: 1 hour

Servings: 4

Ginger powder is stacked with clinical benefits, while a curry stick makes your food tastes so amazing. You can moreover add herbed salt, paprika, chives, and other zing blends.

Per serving:

- 295 Calories;
- 19.5g Fat;
- 2.9g Carbs;
- 25.5g Protein;
- 3.1g Sugars

Fixings:

- 4 teaspoons sesame oil
- 1 pound turkey wings, boneless and chopped
- 2 cloves garlic, finely chopped
- 1 small-sized red chili pepper, minced
- 1/2 teaspoon turmeric powder
- 1/2 teaspoon ginger powder
- 1 teaspoon red curry paste
- 1 cup unsweetened coconut milk, preferably homemade
- 1/2 cup water
- 1/2 cup turkey consommé Kosher salt and ground black pepper, to taste

Headings

Heat sesame oil in a sauté skillet. Add the turkey and cook until it is light brown around 7 minutes.

Add garlic, bean stew pepper, turmeric powder, ginger powder, and curry paste and cook for 3 minutes longer.

Add the milk, water, and consommé. Season with salt and dim pepper. Cook for 45 minutes over medium hotness. Bon appétit!

12. RANCH CHICKEN BREASTS WITH CHEESE

Prepared in around: 20 minutes

Servings: 4

Per serving:

- 295 Calories;
- 19.5g Fat;
- 2.9g Carbs;
- 25.5g Protein;
- 3.1g Sugars

Fixings:

- 2 chicken breasts
- 2 tablespoons butter, melted
- 1 teaspoon salt
- 1/2 teaspoon garlic powder
- 1/2 teaspoon cayenne pepper
- 1/2 teaspoon black peppercorns, crushed
- 1/2 tablespoon ranch seasoning mix
- 4 ounces Ricotta cheese, room temperature
- 1/2 cup Monterey-Jack cheese, grated
- 4 slices bacon, chopped
- 1/4 cup scallions, chopped

Headings

Start by preheating your oven to 370 degrees F.

Give the chicken condensed margarine. Rub the chicken with salt, garlic powder, cayenne pepper, dim pepper, and homestead getting ready mix.

Heat a cast iron skillet over medium hotness. Cook the chicken for 3 to 5 minutes for each side. Move the chicken to a delicately lubed baking dish.

Add cheddar and bacon. Plan around 12 minutes. Top with scallions not long before serving. Bon appétit!

13. CHEESY CHICKEN DRUMSTICKS

Prepared in around: 20 minutes

Servings: 2

Chicken, flavors, and lots of cheddar... what's not to venerate about these low-carb, smooth drumsticks? Nut oil has a high smoke point; you can use rough sunflower oil and avocado oil, also.

Per serving:

- 589 Calories;
- 46g Fat;
- 5.8g Carbs;
- 1g Fiber;
- 37.5g Protein;
- 3.8g Sugars

Fixings:

- 1 tablespoon peanut oil
- 2 chicken drumsticks
- 1/2 cup vegetable broth
- 1/2 cup cream cheese
- 2 cups baby spinach Sea salt and ground black pepper, to taste
- 1/2 teaspoon parsley flakes
- 1/2 teaspoon shallot powder
- 1/2 teaspoon garlic powder
- 1/2 cup Asiago cheese, grated

Headings

Heat the oil in a dish over medium-high hotness. Then, cook the chicken for 7 minutes, turning rarely; save.

Pour in stock; add cream cheddar and spinach; cook until spinach has wilted. Add the chicken back to the dish.

Add flavors and Asiago cheddar; cook until everything is totally warmed, an additional 4 minutes. Serve rapidly and appreciate!

14. UNCOMMON CHICKEN SALAD

Prepared in around: 1 hour 20 minutes

Servings: 3

You can add foamed eggs to the plate of leafy greens a lot of like grandmas used to make. You can moreover use additional chicken from a feast chicken.

Per serving:

- 400 Calories;
- 35.1g Fat;
- 5.6g Carbs;
- 2.9g Fiber;
- 16.1g Protein;
- 2.2g Sugars

Fixings:

- 1 chicken breast, skinless
- 1/4 mayonnaise
- 1/4 cup sour cream
- 2 tablespoons Cottage cheese, room temperature Salt and black pepper, to taste
- 1/4 cup sunflower seeds, hulled and roasted
- 1/2 avocado, peeled and cubed
- 1/2 teaspoon fresh garlic, minced
- 2 tablespoons scallions, chopped

Headings

Bring a pot of all around salted water to a moving air pocket.

Add the chicken to the foaming water; as of now, switch off the hotness, cover, and let the chicken substitute the warmed water for 15 minutes.

Then, channel the water; hack the chicken into downsized pieces. Add the extra trimmings and mix well.

Place in the refrigerator for somewhere near an hour. Function admirably for chilled. Appreciate!

15. TURKEY CRUST PIZZA WITH BACON

Prepared in around: 35 minutes

Servings: 4

This tasty low-carb pizza is far better than takeout. Other fixing considerations fuse pepperoni, spinach, onion, and marinara sauce. Appreciate!

Per serving:

- 360 Calories;
- 22.7g Fat;
- 5.9g Carbs;
- 0.7g Fiber;
- 32.6g Protein;
- 2.7g Sugars

Fixings:

- 1/2-pound ground turkey
- 1/2 cup Parmesan cheese, freshly grated
- 1/2 cup Mozzarella cheese grated Salt and ground black pepper, to taste
- 1 bell pepper, sliced
- 2 slices Canadian bacon, chopped
- 1 tomato, chopped
- 1 teaspoon oregano
- 1/2 teaspoon basil

Headings

In mixing bowl, totally combine the ground turkey, cheddar, salt, and dull pepper.

Then, press the cheddar chicken mix into a material lined baking dish. Plan in the preheated oven, at 390 degrees F for 22 minutes.

Add ring pepper, bacon, tomato, oregano, and basil. Plan an additional 10 minutes and serve warm. Bon appétit!

16. OUTDATED CHICKEN SOUP

Prepared in around: 55 minutes

Servings: 6

This no-noodle chicken soup is great and delicious when it's cold outside. It will be a huge hit all through the colder season!

Per serving:

- 265 Calories;
- 23.8g Fat;
- 4.3g Carbs;
- 1.7g Fiber;
- 9.3g Protein;
- 2.3g Sugars

Fixings:

- 1 rotisserie chicken, shredded
- 6 cups water
- 2 tablespoons butter.
- 3 celery stalks, chopped
- 1/2 onion, chopped
- 1 bay leaf Sea salt and ground black pepper, to taste
- 1 tablespoon fresh cilantro, chopped
- 2 cups green cabbage, sliced into strips

Headings

Cook the bones and carcass from an additional a chicken with water over medium-high hotness for 15 minutes. Then, abatement to a stew and cook an additional 15 minutes. Save the chicken close by the stock.

Permit it to adequately cool to manage, shred the meat into downsized pieces. Break down the spread in a colossal stockpot over medium hotness. Sauté the celery and onion until sensitive and fragrant.

Add sound leaf, salt, pepper, and stock, and let it stew for 10 minutes.

Add the saved chicken, cilantro, and cabbage. Stew for an additional a 10 to 11 minutes, until the cabbage is sensitive. Bon appétit!

17. FIRM CHICKEN FILETS IN TOMATO SAUCE

Prepared in around: 15 minutes

Servings: 3

The way in to this equation is to crush the pork skins in a Ziploc sack the most difficult way possible, since we truly need a panko-like surface. An essential pureed tomato comes very well with chicken.

Per serving:

- 359 Calories;
- 23.6g Fat;
- 5.8g Carbs;
- 1.2g Fiber;
- 30.4g Protein;
- 3.1g Sugars

Fixings:

- 1 tablespoon double cream
- 1 egg
- 2 ounces pork rinds, crushed
- 2 ounces Romano cheese, grated Sea salt and ground black pepper, to taste
- 1 teaspoon cayenne pepper
- 1 teaspoon dried parsley
- 1 garlic clove, halved
- 1/2-pound chicken fillets
- 3 tablespoons olive oil
- 1 large-sized Roma tomato, pureed

Heading

In a mixing bowl, whisk the cream and egg.

In another bowl, mix the crushed pork skins, Romano cheddar, salt, dim pepper, cayenne pepper, and dried parsley.

Rub the garlic parts generally the chicken. Dive the chicken filets into the egg blend; then, cover the chicken with breading on all sides.

Heat the olive oil in a compartment over medium-high hotness; add ghee. Once hot, cook chicken filets until by and by not pink, 2 to 4 minutes on each side.

Move the coordinated chicken filets to a baking dish that is delicately lubed with a nonstick cooking sprinkle. Cover with the pureed tomato. Get ready for 2 to 3 minutes until everything is totally warmed. Bon appétit!

18. LEMON GARLIC GRILLED CHICKEN WINGS

Prepared in around: 25 minutes + marinating time

Servings: 4

For a quick dinner on involved weeknights, place a couple of chicken wings and marinade in a Ziploc pack; hold up them and voila! For a genuine day, thaw out them and set on the preheated grill.

Per serving:

- 131 Calories;
- 7.8g Fat;
- 1.8g Carbs;
- 0.2g Fiber;
- 13.4g Protein;
- 0.4g Sugars

Fixings:

- 8 chicken wings
- 2 tablespoons ghee, melted The Marinade:
- 2 garlic cloves, minced
- 1/4 cup leeks, chopped
- 2 tablespoons lemon juice Salt and ground black pepper, to taste
- 1/2 teaspoon paprika
- 1 teaspoon dried rosemary

Headings

Totally join all components for the marinade in an earth bowl. Add the chicken wings to the bowl.

Cover and license it to marinate for an hour.

Then, preheat your grill to medium-high hotness. Sprinkle melted ghee over the chicken wings. Grill the chicken wings for 20 minutes, turning them at times.

Taste, change the flavors, and serve warm. Appreciate!

PORK

19. MEXICAN-STYLE PORK TACOS

Prepared in around: 20 minutes

Servings: 4

You could serve this pork mix on a bed of zucchini noodles. Other popular decorations fuse obliterated cheddar, guacamole, Tabasco sauce, mustard, tomato, and ringer peppers.

Per serving:

- 330 Calories;
- 26.3g Fat;
- 4.9g Carbs;
- 1.3g Fiber;
- 17.9g Protein;
- 2.4g Sugars

Fixings:

- 1 ounce's ground pork
- 4 ounces ground turkey Sea salt and ground black pepper, to taste
- 1 tablespoon lard
- 4 tablespoons roasted tomatillo salsa
- 12 lettuce leaves
- 4 tablespoons fresh cilantro, chopped
- 4 tablespoons sour cream

Headings

In a mixing bowl, totally combine the ground pork, turkey, salt, and dull pepper. Break up the fat in a skillet over medium-high hotness. Once hot, cook the meat mix for 5 to 6 minutes, deteriorating with a fork.

Add the seared tomatillo salsa and blend to solidify well.

To accumulate the tacos, parcel the salsa-meat mix between lettuce leaves. Top with cilantro and bitter cream. Make wraps and serve immediately.

20. PORK CUTLETS IN CHILI TANGY SAUCE

Prepared in around: 15 minutes

Servings: 4

These pork cutlets are perfectly ready and cooked with piles of flavors. Finally, they are given a hot sherry sauce.

Per serving:

- 288 Calories;
- 17.3g Fat;
- 1.1g Carbs;
- 29.9g Protein;
- 0.1g Sugars

Fixings:

- 1 pound pork cutlets Sea salt and ground black pepper, to taste
- 1/2 teaspoon thyme
- 1/2 teaspoon rosemary
- 1 teaspoon basil
- 1 tablespoon lard, room temperature
- The Sauce: 1 tablespoons sherry
- 1/4 cup sour cream
- 1/4 cup beef bone broth
- 1 teaspoon mustard
- 1/2 teaspoon turmeric powder
- 1/2 teaspoon chili powder

Headings

Season the pork cutlets with salt, pepper, thyme, rosemary, and basil.

Break down the fat in a dish over medium-high hotness; by and by, scorch pork cutlets for 3 minutes; turn them over and cook for 3 minutes on the contrary side. Hold.

Deglaze your skillet with sherry; as of now, add the overabundance trimmings and cook on medium-low hotness until the sauce has thickened insignificantly. Add the saved pork and let it stew for quite a long time or until everything is warmed through. Spoon the sauce over pork cutlets and serve.

21. EVENT PORK BELLY WITH VEGETABLES

Prepared in around: 20 minutes

Servings: 4

Would it be able to be said that you are contemplating an oven stewed firm pork? Look no further! This pork stomach is fragile with shocking new skin.

Per serving:

- 607 Calories;
- 60g Fat;
- 4.4g Carbs;
- 0.7g Fiber;
- 11.4g Protein;
- 2.1g Sugars

Fixings:

- 1-pound skinless pork belly Himalayan salt and freshly ground black pepper, to taste
- 1 teaspoon dried parsley
- 1 teaspoon dried basil
- 1/2 teaspoon dried oregano
- 2 cloves garlic, pressed
- 1/2 cup shallots, sliced
- 1 red bell pepper, seeded and sliced
- 1 green bell pepper, seeded and sliced

Headings

Poke holes all around the pork with a fork. Rub the flavors all around the pork midriff. Place the pork in a tenderly lubed baking skillet.

Top with garlic, shallots, and peppers. Move the pork midriff to the preheated grill.

Heat at 390 degrees F for around 18 minutes. Serve warm.

22. CHEESEBURGER SKILLET WITH BACON AND MUSHROOMS

Prepared in around: 20 minutes

Servings: 4

Would it be able to be said that you are craving cheeseburgers anyway you don't have the potential chance to cook them? No worries, this surprising dish gets together in one skillet in less than 20 minutes.

Per serving:

- 463 Calories;
- 60g Fat;
- 4.7g Carbs;
- 0.8g Fiber;
- 36.2g Protein;
- 3g Sugars

Fixings:

- 1 slice Canadian bacon, chopped
- 1/2 cup shallots, sliced
- 1 garlic clove, minced
- 1 pound ground pork Sea salt and ground black pepper, to taste
- 1/3 cup vegetable broth
- 1/4 cup white wine
- 6 ounces Cremini mushrooms, sliced
- 1/2 cup cream cheese

Headings

Heat a cast-iron skillet over medium hotness. Cook the bacon for 2 to 3 minutes; save the bacon and 1 tablespoon of fat. Then, sauté the shallots and garlic in 1 tablespoon of bacon fat until fragile and fragrant.

Add the ground pork, salt, and dim pepper to the skillet. Cook for 4 to 5 minutes or until ground meat is well caramelized.

Add stock, wine, and mushrooms. Cover and cook for 8 to 9 minutes over medium fire. Switch off the hotness. Add cream cheddar and blend to join. Serve polished off with the held bacon. Appreciate!

23. COUNTRY-STYLE PORK STEW

Prepared in around: 40 minutes

Servings: 4

Per serving:

- 351 Calories;
- 22.7g Fat;
- 2.7g Carbs;
- 0.5g Fiber;
- 32.3g Protein;
- 1.5g Sugars

Fixings:

- 2 tablespoons lard, room temperature
- 1/4 cup leeks, chopped
- 3 garlic cloves, minced
- 1 (1-inch) piece ginger root, peeled and chopped
- 1 bell pepper, seeded and chopped
- 1 pound pork stew meat, cubed
- 1/2 cup tomato paste
- 2 cups chicken broth Sea salt and ground black pepper, to taste
- 1 teaspoon paprika
- 1 bay leaf
- 1/4 cup Crème fraiche

Headings

Break down the fat in a sauté compartment that is preheated over medium hotness. Then, cook the leeks, garlic, and ginger until fragrant, around 3 minutes.

Add ring pepper and cook for a further 2 minutes, blending sometimes. Add the pork and cook an additional 3 minutes or until as of now not pink.

Blend in the tomato stick, stock, salt, pepper, paprika, and strait leaf. Cover and let it stew over low-medium hotness around 30 minutes.

Blend in Crème fraiche; switch off the hotness and blend until everything is generally merged. Scoop into serving bowls and serve immediately.

24. MUDDLED AND BUTTERY PORK CHOPS

Prepared in around: 20 minutes

Servings: 2

If you are in a hurry, these pork hacks with cheddar, flavors and spread are faster than mentioning takeout. You can use any full-fat, firm cheddar of your choice.

Per serving:

- 494 Calories;
- 39.8g Fat;
- 5.3g Carbs;
- 1.1g Fiber;
- 28.6g Protein;
- 2.7g Sugars

Fixings:

- 1/2 stick butter, room temperature
- 1/2 cup white onion, chopped
- 4 ounces button mushrooms, sliced
- 1/3-pound pork loin chops
- 1 teaspoon dried parsley flakes Salt and ground black pepper, to taste
- 1/2 cup Swiss cheese, shredded

Headings

Relax 1/4 of the spread stick in a skillet over medium hotness. Then, sauté the onions and mushrooms until the onions are clear and the mushrooms are sensitive and fragrant, around 5 minutes. Save.

Then, relax the extra 1/4 of the spread stick and cook pork until insignificantly sautéed on all sides, around 10 minutes.

Add the onion blend, parsley, salt, and pepper. Eventually, top with cheddar; cover and let it cook on medium-low hotness until cheddar has disintegrated. Serve instantly and appreciate!

25. FILIPINO NILAGA SOUP

Prepared in around: 45 minutes

Servings: 4

You can use a languid cooker to cook this soup; cook on high for 4 hours or until the meat is fork-fragile. You can similarly add cheeseburger heave dinner or ribs and cook it all together.

Per serving:

- 203 Calories;
- 8.4g Fat;
- 3.7g Carbs;
- 1.1g Fiber;
- 27.1g Protein;
- 1.7g Sugars

Fixings:

- 1 teaspoon butter
- 1 pound pork ribs, boneless and cut into small pieces
- 1 shallot, chopped
- 2 garlic cloves, minced
- 1 (1/2-inch) piece fresh ginger, chopped
- 1 cup water 2 cups chicken stock
- 1 tablespoon pates (fish sauce)
- 1 cup fresh tomatoes, pureed
- 1 cup cauliflower "rice" Sea salt and ground black pepper, to taste

Headings

Relax the spread in a pot over medium-high hotness. Then, cook the pork ribs on all sides for 5 to 6 minutes.

Add the shallot, garlic and ginger; cook an additional 3 minutes. Add the abundance trimmings.

Permit it to cook, covered, for 30 to 35 minutes. Scoop into individual dishes and serve.

26. PORK TENDERLOIN WITH SOUTHERN CABBAGE

Prepared in around: 25 minutes

Servings: 2

You can marinate pork for safe tenderloin at whatever point needed. Capable cooks add a dash of lemon juice to the cabbage while cooking.

Per serving:

- 254 Calories;
- 10.8g Fat;
- 5.7g Carbs;
- 1.6g Fiber;
- 31.8g Protein;
- 3.3g Sugars

Fixings:

The Pork tenderloin:

- 1/2-pound pork tenderloin Celtic Sea salt and freshly cracked black pepper, to taste
- 1/2 teaspoon granulated garlic
- 1/4 teaspoon ginger powder
- 1/2 teaspoon dried sage
- 1 tablespoon lard, room temperature

The Cabbage:

- 5 ounces cabbage, sliced into strips
- 1/3 cup vegetable broth 2 tablespoons sherry wine
- 1/2 teaspoon mustard seeds Celtic Sea salt, to taste
- 1/2 teaspoon black peppercorns

Headings

Season the pork with salt, dull pepper, granulated garlic, ginger powder, and sage.

Condense the oil in a dish over moderate hotness. Sear the pork for 7 to 8 minutes, turning irregularly.

In a compartment that is preheated over medium hotness, bring the cabbage, stock, sherry, and mustard seeds to an air pocket over high hotness. Season with salt and dull peppercorns; cook, mixing at times, until the cabbage is sensitive, around 12 minutes; don't overcook.

Serve the pork with sautéed cabbage as an untimely idea. Bon appétit!

27. INDIAN-STYLE FRIED PORK

Prepared in around: 15 minutes

Servings: 4

Pork shoulder is the best cut for this recipe; it has a remarkable meat to fat extent. Present with crushed cauliflower and you will have an ideal ketogenic, family supper.

Per serving:

- 478 Calories;
- 34.7g Fat;
- 2.2g Carbs;
- 36.4g Protein;
- 0.3g Sugars

Fixings:

- 1 teaspoon shallot powder
- 1 teaspoon porcini powder
- 1 teaspoon garlic powder
- 1/2 teaspoon cumin
- 1/4 teaspoon turmeric powder
- 1 cinnamon stick
- 2 dried Kashmiri red chilies, roasted Sea salt and ground black pepper, to taste
- 1 pound pork shoulder
- 1/2 cup ground pork rinds
- 1/2 cup Parmesan cheese, grated
- 3 eggs
- 2 tablespoons tallow

Headings

Blend the flavors alongside the cinnamon and chilies until you have a smooth paste. Rub this stick all around the pork shoulder. In a bowl, join the pork skins with parmesan cheddar. In an alternate bowl, whisk the eggs. Cut the pork into little pieces; plunge the pork in the egg and a while later, cover it with the pork skin blend. Condense the fat in a skillet over medium-high hotness. Cook the pork for 2 to 3 minutes for each side. Bon appétit!

MEAT

28. ITALIAN-STYLE SPICY MEATBALLS

Prepared in around: 15 minutes

Servings: 3

Is it genuine that you are in the demeanor for meatballs? Participate in all of the brilliant sorts of Italian cooking in these lively and chaotic meatballs.

Per serving:

- 458 Calories;
- 35.8g Fat;
- 4.3g Carbs;
- 0.2g Fiber;
- 28.2g Protein;
- 3.1g Sugars

Fixings:

Sauce:

- 4 ounces Asiago cheese, grated
- 1/4 cup mayonnaise
- 1 chili pepper, minced
- 1 teaspoon yellow mustard
- 1 teaspoon Italian parsley
- 1/2 teaspoon red pepper flakes, crushed
- 1/2 teaspoon sea salt
- 1/2 teaspoon ground black pepper

Meatballs:

- 1/2-pound ground beef
- 1 egg
- 1 tablespoon olive oil

Headings

In a bowl, totally combine the cheddar, mayo, stew, mustard, parsley, red pepper, salt, and dim pepper.

Then, blend in the ground meat and egg. Blend to combine well. Shape the mix into meatballs.

By and by, heat the oil in a skillet over a moderate fire. Once hot, cook the meatballs for 2 to 3 minutes on each side. Serve and appreciate!

29. RICH DOUBLE-CHEESE MEATLOAF

Prepared in around: 1 hour

Servings: 4

This is the best blend of delectableness and comfort. It's truly brilliant for the accompanying event.

Per serving:

- 361 Calories;
- 23.1g Fat;
- 5.6g Carbs;
- 0.8g Fiber;
- 32.2g Protein;
- 2.5g Sugars

Fixings:

- 1 teaspoon sunflower oil
- 1/2 cup onions, chopped
- 2 cloves garlic, minced
- 1 bell pepper, seeded and chopped
- 1 jalapeno pepper, seeded and chopped
- 3/4-pound ground beef
- 1/4-pound bacon, chopped
- 1/2 Swiss cheese, grated
- 1/2 cup Parmesan cheese, grated
- 1 egg, whisked
- 1 teaspoon oyster sauce Sea salt and ground black pepper, to taste
- 1 ripe tomato, pureed
- 1 teaspoon Dijon mustard

Headings

Start by preheating your grill to 390 degrees F. Delicately oil a baking holder with a nonstick cooking sprinkle.

Heat the oil in a holder over a moderate fire. By and by, sauté the onions, garlic, and peppers until sensitive and sweet-smelling, around 5 minutes.

In a mixing bowl, totally join the ground meat, bacon, cheddar, egg, shellfish sauce, salt, and ground dim pepper. Structure the blend into a piece and press it into the baking compartment; spread the mix of pureed tomato and mustard over the top.

Cover the dish with foil and hotness for 50 minutes in the preheated oven.

Appreciate!

30. MEAT AND GOAT CHEESE STUFFED MUSHROOMS

Prepared in around: 25 minutes

Servings: 5

You can serve these mushrooms as the ideal enhancement to any keto dinner or an absolute supper, it's subject to you. In less than 25 minutes you can have a phenomenal dish that everyone loves.

Per serving:

- 148 Calories;
- 8.4g Fat;
- 4.8g Carbs;
- 1.1g Fiber;
- 14.1g Protein;
- 2.7g Sugars

Fixings:

- 3 ounces ground beef
- 2 ounces ground pork Kosher salt and ground black pepper, to taste
- 1/4 cup goat cheese, crumbled
- 2 tablespoons Romano cheese, grated
- 2 tablespoons shallot, minced
- 1 garlic clove, minced
- 1 teaspoon dried basil
- 1/2 teaspoon dried oregano
- 1/2 teaspoon dried rosemary
- 20 button mushrooms, stems removed

Headings

Solidify all trimmings, except for the mushrooms, in a mixing bowl. Then, stuff the mushrooms with this filling.

Get ready in the preheated oven at 370 degrees F around 18 minutes. Serve warm or cold. Bon appétit!

31. OBLITERATED BEEF WITH HERBS

Prepared in around: 50 minutes

Servings: 4

Make a pass at something legitimate and make this dish for the accompanying family collecting! Serve obliterated meat over keto tacos or cauliflower rice.

Per serving:

- 421 Calories;
- 35.7g Fat;
- 5.9g Carbs;
- 1g Fiber;
- 19.7g Protein;
- 2.7g Sugars

Fixings:

- 1 tablespoon olive oil
- 1 pound rib eye, cut into strips
- 2 tablespoons rice wine
- 1/4 cup beef bone broth Sea salt and ground black pepper, to taste
- 2 tablespoons fresh parsley, finely chopped
- 2 tablespoons fresh chives, finely chopped
- 2 chipotle peppers in adobo sauce, chopped
- 1 garlic clove, crushed
- 2 small-sized ripe tomatoes, pureed
- 1 yellow onion, peeled and chopped
- 1/2 teaspoon dry mustard
- 1 teaspoon dried basil
- 1 teaspoon dried marjoram

Headings

Heat the oil in a dish over medium-high hotness. Scorch the meat for 6 to 7 minutes, mixing incidentally. Work in gatherings.

Add the extra trimmings, decrease the hotness to medium-low and let it cook for 40 minutes.

Shred the meat and serve. Bon appétit!

32. CHINESE GROUND BEEF SKILLET

Prepared in around: 15 minutes

Servings: 3

Right when you extreme a burger dish burns with Asian flavors, endeavor this equation. The basic trimmings to the best Chinese food fuse soy sauce, rice wine, and natural shaded mushrooms.

Per serving:

- 179 Calories;
- 10.4g Fat;
- 5.8g Carbs;
- 1g Fiber;
- 16.5g Protein;
- 2.6g Sugars

Fixings:

- 1 tablespoon sesame oil
- 1/2-pound ground chuck
- 1 shallot, minced
- 1 garlic clove, minced
- 1 (1/2-inch) piece ginger root, peeled and grated
- 1 bell pepper, seeded and sliced
- 4 ounces brown mushrooms, sliced
- 1 teaspoon tamari soy sauce
- 1 tablespoon rice wine
- 2 whole star anise Himalayan salt and ground black pepper, to taste

Headings

Heat the oil in a skillet over a moderate fire. By and by, cook the ground throw until it is now not pink. Save.

Then, cook the shallot, garlic, ginger, pepper, and mushrooms in skillet drippings. Add the abundance trimmings close by held meat to the holder.

Reduce the hotness to medium-low; let it stew for 2 to 3 minutes longer. Attempt to blend incessantly. Appreciate!

33. BASIC STEAK SALAD

Prepared in around: 20 minutes

Servings: 4

At times you essentially need a clear plate of leafy greens for lunch. You can make an awesome keto salad start to finish in less than 20 minutes.

Per serving:

- 231 Calories;
- 17.1g Fat;
- 6g Carbs;
- 3.4g Fiber;
- 13.8g Protein;
- 1.5g Sugars

Fixings:

- 1 tablespoons olive oil
- 8 ounces flank steak, salt-and-pepper-seasoned
- 1 cucumber, sliced
- 1/2 cup onions finely sliced.
- 1 ripe avocado, peeled and sliced
- 2 medium-sized heirloom tomatoes, sliced
- 3 ounces baby arugula
- 1 tablespoon fresh coriander, chopped
- 4 tablespoons lime juice

Headings

Heat 1 tablespoon of olive oil in a dish over medium-high hotness. Cook the flank steak for 5 minutes, turning a couple of times.

Let address 10 minutes; then, cut gently across the grain. Move the meat to a bowl.

Add cucumbers, shallots, avocado, tomatoes, youngster arugula, and new coriander. As of now, shower your plate of leafy greens with lime juice and the extra 1 tablespoon of olive oil.

Function admirably for chilled and appreciate!

34. CHEEKY SKIRT STEAK WITH BROCCOLI

Prepared in around: 15 minutes + marinating time

Servings: 3

Broccoli is the ideal fixing when we need a little a reward to adjust our keto supper. Other than being delightful, broccoli enjoys various health advantages.

Per serving:

- 31 Calories;
- 24.7g Fat;
- 4.5g Carbs;
- 2.8g Fiber;
- 24.1g Protein;
- 0.9g Sugars

Fixings:

- 1/2-pound skirt steak, sliced into pieces
- 2 tablespoons butter, room temperature
- 1/2-pound broccoli, cut into florets
- 1/2 cup scallions, chopped
- 1 clove garlic, pressed

Marinade:

- 1/2 teaspoon ground black pepper
- 1 teaspoon red pepper flakes
- 1/2 teaspoon sea salt
- 2 tablespoons olive oil
- 1 tablespoon tamari sauce
- 1/4 cup wine vinegar

Headings

In a pottery bowl totally merge all components for the marinade. Add the cheeseburger and license it to sit in your cooler for 2 hours.

Mellow 1 tablespoon of spread in a skillet over high to medium-high hotness. Cook the broccoli for 2 minutes, mixing frequently, until it is sensitive anyway stunning green.

Condense the abundance tablespoon of spread in the skillet. Once hot, cook the scallions and garlic until fragrant, around 2 minutes. Hold.

Then, at that point, consume the meat, adding an unobtrusive amount of the marinade. Cook until a lot of singed on all sides or around 10 minutes.

Add the saved vegetables and cook for a few minutes more or until everything is warmed through. Bon appétit!

35. MODEL BEEF STROGANOFF

Prepared in around: 1 hour

Servings: 4

Burger stew meat is clearer to cut in case it's fairly frozen. Sautéing the garlic and onion will help with portraying their clever taste anyway you can skirt this movement accepting you are in a hurry.

Per serving:

- 303 Calories;
- 17.2g Fat;
- 5.6g Carbs;
- 0.9g Fiber;
- 32.4g Protein;
- 1.8g Sugars

Fixings:

- 2 tablespoons lard, room temperature
- 1 pound beef stew meat, cut across grain into strips
- 1/2 yellow onion, peeled and chopped
- 2 garlic cloves, minced
- 5 ounces fresh mushrooms, sliced
- 1/2 teaspoon salt
- 1 teaspoon smoked paprika
- 1/4 teaspoon black pepper
- 1/2 teaspoon dried basil
- 1/4 cup red cooking wine
- 4 cups vegetable broth
- 1 fresh tomato, pureed
- 2 celery stalks, chopped
- 1/2 cup sour cream

Headings

Mellow the oil in a stockpot over medium hotness. Then, cook the meat until well caramelized on all sides.

Then, add onion and garlic and cook until they are fragrant. By and by, blend in the mushrooms and cook until they are sensitive.

Add flavors, wine, stock, tomato, and celery. Decrease hotness, cover, and stew for 50 minutes.

Switch off the hotness and add brutal cream; blend until warmed through.

Taste, change the flavors, and serve warm. Bon appétit!

FISH and SEAFOOD

36. CATFISH AND CAULIFLOWER CASSEROLE

Prepared in around: 30 minutes

Servings: 4

New aromatics and dried flavors give this fish goulash an extra extraordinary taste. Your family will demand more!

Per serving:

- 510 Calories;
- 40g Fat;
- 5.5g Carbs;
- 1.6g Fiber;
- 31.3g Protein;
- 3g Sugars

Fixings:

- 1 tablespoon sesame oil
- 11 ounces cauliflower
- 4 scallions
- 1 garlic clove, minced
- 1 teaspoon fresh ginger root, grated Salt and ground black pepper, to taste Cayenne pepper, to taste
- 2 sprigs dried thyme, crushed
- 1 sprig rosemary, crushed
- 24 ounces catfish, cut into pieces
- 1/2 cup cream cheese
- 1/2 cup double cream
- 1 egg
- 2 ounces butter, cold

Headings

Start by preheating your grill to 390 degrees F. As of now, delicately oil a feast dish with a nonstick cooking shower.

Then, heat the oil in a skillet over medium-high hotness; once hot, cook the cauliflower and scallions until sensitive or 5 to 6 minutes. Add the garlic and ginger; continue to sauté brief more.

Move the vegetables to the set-up goulash dish. Sprinkle with flavors. Add catfish to the top.

In a mixing bowl, totally join the cream cheddar, twofold cream, and egg. Spread this smooth mix over the most noteworthy place of your feast.

Top with cuts of spread. Get ready in the preheated oven for 18 to 22 minutes or until the fish drops successfully with a fork. Bon appétit!

37. SWEDISH HERRING SALAD

Prepared in around: 10 minutes

Servings: 3

I made this plate of leafy greens following encountering energetic affections for Upstreaming (Swedish for a gently salted developed Baltic Sea herring). This makes an ideal event salad moreover.

Per serving:

- 134 Calories;
- 7.9g Fat;
- 5.4g Carbs;
- 1g Fiber;
- 10.2g Protein;
- 2.3g Sugars

Fixings:

- 5 ounces pickled herring pieces, drained and flaked
- 1/2 cup baby spinach
- 3 tablespoons fresh basil leaves
- 3 tablespoons fresh chives, chopped
- 1 teaspoon garlic, minced
- 1 bell pepper, chopped
- 1 red onion, chopped
- 2 tablespoons key lime juice, freshly squeezed Sea salt and ground black pepper, to taste

Headings

In a plate of leafy greens bowl solidify the herring pieces with spinach, basil leaves, chives, garlic, ringer pepper, and red onion.

Then, shower key lime juice over the plate of leafy greens; add salt and pepper to taste and toss to join. Smalling malted! Bon appétit!

38. GREAT FISHERMAN'S STEW

Prepared in around: 30 minutes

Servings: 4

Endeavor a top pick equation for a fish stew with a Mediterranean reshape! You can use frozen or new trimmings; at any rate, it will taste extraordinary.

Per serving:

- 271 Calories;
- 19.5g Fat;
- 4.8g Carbs;
- 1g Fiber;
- 18.5g Protein;
- 1.3g Sugars

Fixings:

- 1 tablespoon tallow, room temperature
- 1 red onion, chopped
- 2 garlic cloves, smashed
- 1 jalapeno pepper, chopped
- 1/2 bunch fresh dill, roughly chopped
- 1 ripe fresh tomato, pureed
- 1 cup shellfish stock
- 3 cups water
- 1 pound halibut, cut into bite-sized chunks Sea salt and ground black pepper, to taste
- 1 teaspoon cayenne pepper
- 1/2 teaspoon curry powder
- 2 bay leaves

Headings

Disintegrate the fat in a colossal pot over medium-high hotness. Then, sweat the onion for 3 minutes; blend in the garlic and jalapeno pepper and sauté brief more. Add new dill and tomato; cook for 8 minutes more. Pour in shellfish stock and water. Add salt, dim pepper, cayenne pepper, curry powder, and sound leaves. Reduction to a stew; cook until everything is totally cooked or for 15 minutes.

39. FISH AND VEGETABLE MEDLEY

Prepared in around: 20 minutes

Servings: 4

Cod may override the snapper, and other keto veggies may be used, for instance, green beans or ringer peppers. Snapper is a lean wellspring of protein that is stacked with vitamin A, potassium, omega-3 unsaturated fats, and basic minerals.

Per serving:

- 151 Calories;
- 3g Fat;
- 5.8g Carbs;
- 1.5g Fiber;
- 24.4g Protein;
- 2.8g Sugars

Fixings:

- 1 teaspoon sesame oil
- 1/2 cup scallions, thinly sliced
- 1/2 teaspoon fresh ginger, grated
- 1/2 teaspoon garlic, crushed
- 1 teaspoon red curry paste
- 3 whole star anise
- 1 teaspoon smoked paprika
- 2 ripe tomatoes crushed Coarse Sea salt and ground black pepper, to taste
- 1 pound snapper, cut into bite-sized pieces

Headings

Heat the oil in a pot over moderate hotness. Cook the scallion until fragile and sweet-smelling; by and by, add ginger and garlic and cook an additional 40 seconds, mixing a large part of the time.

Add the overabundance trimmings and lessen the hotness to medium-low. Permit it to stew for 15 minutes or until the fish pieces adequately with a fork. Bon appétit!

40. SALMON CURRY WITH A TWIST

Prepared in around: 20 minutes

Servings: 4

Concerning flavors, certain people don't incline toward strong flavors, as they like to keep the salmon flavor winning. You can similarly add garam masala and ginger-garlic paste to this curry.

Per serving:

- 246 Calories;
- 16.2g Fat;
- 4.9g Carbs;
- 0.6g Fiber;
- 20.3g Protein;
- 2.1g Sugars

Fixings:

- 1 tablespoon coconut oil
- 1/2 cup leeks, chopped
- 1 teaspoon garlic, smashed
- 1 Thai chili pepper, seeded and minced
- 1 teaspoon turmeric powder
- 1/2 teaspoon cumin
- 4 ounces double cream
- 2 ounces full-fat coconut milk, canned
- 1 cup fish stock
- 1 cup water
- 3/4-pound salmon, cut into bite-sized chunks Salt and ground black pepper, to taste
- 1/4 cup fresh cilantro, roughly chopped

Headings

Heat the oil in a stockpot over medium-high hotness. By and by, sauté the leeks and garlic for 2 to 3 minutes, blending regularly.

Add stew pepper, turmeric, and cumin; cook an additional a second. Add cream, coconut milk, fish stock, water, salmon, salt, and dull pepper.

Decline the hotness and let it stew approximately 12 minutes.

In this way, spoon into individual dishes; serve polished off with new cilantro leaves and appreciate!

41. FISH, AVOCADO AND HAM WRAPS

Prepared in around: 10 minutes + chilling time

Servings: 3

Ahi fish also called yellowfin fish is one of the most adored keto food assortments since it is an eating routine pleasing and stacked with protein. It is stacked with selenium, phosphorus, potassium, vitamin D, and vitamin B-12.

Per serving:

- 308 Calories;
- 19.9g Fat;
- 4.3g Carbs;
- 2.5g Fiber;
- 27.8g Protein;
- 0.8g Sugars

Fixings:

- 1/2 cup dry white wine
- 1/2 cup water
- 1/2 teaspoon mixed peppercorns
- 1/2 teaspoon dry mustard powder
- 1/2-pound ahi tuna steak
- 5 slices of ham
- 1/2 Hass avocado, peeled, pitted and sliced
- 1 tablespoon fresh lemon juice
- 6 lettuce leaves

Headings

Add wine, water, peppercorns, and mustard powder to a skillet and hotness with the eventual result of bubbling. Add the fish and stew carefully for 3 minutes to 5 minutes for each side.

Discard the cooking liquid and cut fish into downsized pieces. Parcel the fish pieces between cuts of ham.

Add avocado and shower with new lemon. Roll the wraps up and place each wrap on a lettuce leaf. Function admirably for chilled. Bon appétit!

42. ALASKAN COD WITH MUSTARD CREAM SAUCE

Prepared in around: 10 minutes

Servings: 4

Alaskan cod filets with mustard cream sauce are a straightforward recipe that passes on the best flavors from typical trimmings. It's unmistakably appropriate for a ketogenic diet.

Per serving:

- 166 Calories;
- 8.2g Fat;
- 2.6g Carbs;
- 0.3g Fiber;
- 19.8g Protein;
- 1.9g Sugars

Fixings:

- 1 tablespoon coconut oil
- 4 Alaskan cod fillets Salt and freshly ground black pepper, to taste
- 5 leaves basil, chiffonade Mustard Cream

Sauce:

- 1 teaspoon yellow mustard
- 1 teaspoon paprika
- 1/4 teaspoon ground bay leaf
- 2 tablespoons cream cheese
- 1/2 cup Greek-style yogurt
- 1 garlic clove, minced
- 1 teaspoon lemon zest
- 1 tablespoon fresh parsley, minced Sea salt and ground black pepper, to taste

Headings

Heat coconut oil in a dish over medium hotness. Sear the fish for 2 to 3 minutes for each side. Season with salt and ground dim pepper.

Mix all components for the sauce until everything is generally joined. Top the fish filets with the sauce and serve enlivened with new basil leaves. Bon appétit!

43. SMOKED HADDOCK FISH BURGERS

Prepared in around: 20 minutes

Servings: 4

The scallions and Parmesan in this basic haddock burger equation pair splendidly with bean stew powder. Serve on keto burger buns, at whatever point needed.

Per serving:

- 174 Calories;
- 11.4g Fat;
- 1.5g Carbs;
- 0.2g Fiber;
- 15.4g Protein;
- 0.3g Sugars

Fixings:

- 1 tablespoon sunflower oil
- 7 ounces smoked haddock
- 1 egg
- 1/4 cup Parmesan cheese, grated
- 1 teaspoon chili powder
- 1 teaspoon dried parsley flakes
- 1/4 cup scallions, chopped
- 1 teaspoon fresh garlic minced Salt and ground black pepper, to taste
- 3 lemon wedges

Headings

Heat 1 tablespoon of oil in a skillet over medium-high hotness. Cook the haddock for 6 minutes or until just cooked through; discard the skin and bones and drop into little pieces.

Mix the smoked haddock, egg, cheddar, bean stew powder, parsley, scallions, garlic, salt, and dim pepper in a tremendous bowl.

Heat the abundance tablespoon of oil and cook fish burgers until they are particularly cooked in the middle or around 6 minutes. Embellish each giving a lemon wedge.

EGGS and DAIRY

44. PAPRIKA OMELET WITH GOAT CHEESE

Prepared in around: 10 minutes

Servings: 2

You can make this go-to omelet every day to stir your absorption. You can use different fillings like bacon, ham, peppers, or spinach. Moreover, breakfast is ready in less than 10 minutes.

Per serving:

- 287 Calories;
- 22.6g Fat;
- 1.3g Carbs;
- 19.8g Protein;
- 1.3g Sugars

Fixings:

- 2 teaspoons ghee, room temperature
- 4 eggs,
- Whisked 4 tablespoons goat cheese
- 1 teaspoon paprika Sea salt and ground black pepper, to taste

Headings

Relax the ghee in a compartment over medium hotness.

Add the whisked eggs to the skillet and cover with the top; decrease the hotness to medium-low.

Cook for 4 minutes; as of now, blend in the cheddar and paprika; continue to cook an additional 3 minutes or until cheddar has mellowed.

Season with salt and pepper and serve immediately. Appreciate!

45. DILLY BOILED EGGS WITH AVOCADO

Prepared in around: 10 minutes

Servings: 3

Nothing beats a masterpiece! The central thing better than foamed eggs is impeccably gurgled eggs given new avocado cuts.

Per serving:

- 222 Calories;
- 17.6g Fat;
- 5.7g Carbs;
- 3.9g Fiber;
- 12.2g Protein;
- 0.9g Sugars

Fixings:

- 6 eggs
- 1/2 teaspoon kosher salt
- 1/2 teaspoon ground black pepper
- 1/2 teaspoon cayenne pepper
- 1/2 teaspoon dried dill weed
- 1 avocado, pitted and sliced
- 1 tablespoon lemon juice

Headings

Place the eggs in a skillet of gurgling water; then, cook over low hotness for 6 minutes.

Strip and separation the eggs. Sprinkle the eggs with salt, dull pepper, cayenne pepper, and dill.

Serve on individual plates; sprinkle the avocado cuts with new lemon crush and present with eggs. Appreciate!

46. GREEK-STYLE FRITTATA WITH HERBS

Prepared in around: 30 minutes

Servings: 4

Mediterranean trimmings make this frittata a morning dinner staple all through the mid-year months. Regardless, you can serve this astonishing dish on any occasion.

Per serving:

- 345 Calories;
- 28.5g Fat;
- 4.4g Carbs;
- 0.6g Fiber;
- 18.2g Protein;
- 2.3g Sugars

Fixings:

- 7 eggs
- 1/2 cup heavy cream
- 3 tablespoons Greek-style yogurt
- 2 ounces bacon, chopped Sea salt and freshly ground black pepper, to taste
- 1 tablespoon olive oil
- 1/2 cup red onions, peeled and sliced
- 1 garlic clove, finely chopped
- 8 Kalamata olives, pitted and sliced
- 1 teaspoon dried oregano
- 1/2 teaspoon dried rosemary
- 1/2 teaspoon dried marjoram
- 4 ounces Feta cheese, crumbled

Headings

Preheat your grill to 360 degrees F. Sprits a baking holder with a nonstick cooking shower.

Mix the eggs, cream, yogurt, bacon, salt, and dim pepper.

Heat the oil in a skillet over medium-high hotness. As of now, cook the onion and garlic until sensitive and fragrant, around 3 minutes. Move the blend to the set-up baking compartment.

Pour the egg blend over the vegetables. Add olives, oregano, rosemary, and marjoram.

Plan about 13 minutes, until the eggs are set. Scatter feta cheddar over the top and hotness an additional 3 minutes. Permit it to sit for 5 minutes; cut into wedges and serve.

47. MANGALOREAN EGG CURRY

Prepared in around: 20 minutes

Servings: 4

Eggs in a hot coconut sauce! Make this delicious mélange of eggs, tomatoes, and southern flavors for lunch or dinner.

Per serving:

- 305 Calories;
- 16.4g Fat;
- 5.7g Carbs;
- 1.1g Fiber;
- 32.2g Protein;
- 4.3g Sugars

Fixings:

- 2 tablespoons rice bran oil
- 1/2 cup scallions, chopped
- 1 teaspoon Kashmiri chili powder
- 1/4 teaspoon carom seeds
- 1/4 teaspoon meth seeds
- Kosher salt and ground black pepper, to taste
- 2 ripe tomatoes, pureed
- 2 teaspoons tamarind paste
- 1/2 cup chicken stock
- 4 boiled eggs, peeled
- 1 teaspoon curry paste
- 2 tablespoons curry leaves
- 1/2 teaspoon cinnamon powder
- 1/2 cup coconut milk
- 1 tablespoon cilantro leaves

Headings

Heat the oil in a dish over medium hotness. By and by, cook the scallions and stew until fragile and fragrant.

Add carom seeds, meth seeds, salt, pepper, and tomatoes; cook for a further 8 minutes.

Then, add the tamarind paste and chicken stock. Decline the hotness to medium-low and cook for 3 minutes more.

Add the eggs, curry stick, curry leaves, cinnamon powder, and coconut milk. Permit it to stew for 6 minutes more. Brighten with cilantro leaves. Bon appétit!

48. EGG, BACON AND KALE MUFFINS

Prepared in around: 25 minutes

Servings: 4

These rolls are ooey-gooey tiny frittatas and they are kid-obliging also. They couldn't be more direct to make!

Per serving:

- 384 Calories;
- 29.8g Fat;
- 5.1g Carbs;
- 1.1g Fiber;
- 24g Protein;
- 2.4g Sugars

Fixings:

- 1/2 cup bacon
- 1 shallot, chopped
- 1 garlic clove, minced
- 1 cup kale
- 1 ripe tomato, chopped
- 6 eggs
- 1 cup Asiago cheese, shredded Salt and black pepper, to taste
- 1 teaspoon dried rosemary
- 1/2 teaspoon dried basil
- 1/2 teaspoon dried marjoram

Headings

Start by preheating your oven to 390 degrees F. Add roll liners to a roll tin.

Preheat your skillet over medium hotness. Cook the bacon for 3 to 4 minutes; by and by, slice the bacon and hold.

By and by, cook the shallots and garlic in the bacon fat until they are fragile. Add the extra trimmings and mix to join well.

Void the player into roll cups and plan for 13 minutes or until the edges are barely caramelized.

License your bread rolls to address 5 minutes before killing from the tin. Bon appétit!

49. MUDDLED BRUSSELS SPROUTS

Prepared in around: 25 minutes

Servings: 4

Brussels sprouts are stacked with vitamin K, fiber, and malignant growth avoidance specialists. Sesame oil is helpful in cutting down glucose levels.

Per serving:

- 202 Calories;
- 16.3g Fat;
- 5.8g Carbs;
- 2.3g Fiber;
- 8.8g Protein;
- 1.9g Sugars

Fixings:

- 3/4-pound Brussels sprouts, cleaned and halved
- 3 tablespoons sesame oil
- 1 teaspoon dried parsley flakes
- 1 sprig dried thyme
- Kosher salt and ground black pepper, to taste
- 7 ounces Colby cheese, shredded

Headings

Start by preheating your oven to 400 degrees F.

Gently oil a baking skillet with a nonstick cooking shower. Arrange the Brussels sprouts on the baking skillet. Sprinkle them with nut oil.

Toss with parsley, thyme, salt, and dim pepper. Cook in the preheated oven around 18 minutes.

Add Colby cheddar and dish an additional 3 minutes. Serve immediately. Appreciate!

50. CAULIFLOWER, CHEESE AND EGG FAT BOMBS

Prepared in around: 35 minutes

Servings: 4

These fat bombs aren't just superb; they're conservative, diet-obliging, and kid-obliging! They merit a spot on your get-away table!

Per serving:

- 168 Calories;
- 10.9g Fat;
- 3.5g Carbs;
- 1.1g Fiber;
- 13.9g Protein;
- 1.4g Sugars

Fixings:

- 1/2-pound cauliflower, cut into florets
- 1/2 cup pork rinds, crushed
- 1/4 cup almond flour
- 1/2 cup Romano cheese, grated
- 2 eggs, beaten

Headings

Heat up the cauliflower until sensitive; channel well. Then, mix the cauliflower in with pork skins, almond flour, Romano cheddar, and eggs; shape the blend into downsized balls.

Arrange the balls in a material lined baking skillet.

Plan in the preheated oven at 345 degrees F around 28 minutes. Serve warm or cold and appreciate!

51. TWOFOLD CHEESE AND SAUSAGE BALLS

Prepared in around: 20 minutes

Servings: 3

It's quite easy to make a tasty keto canapé in less than 20 minutes. If you love breakfast wiener and cheddar, this is the best snack for you!

Per serving:

- 412 Calories;
- 34.6g Fat;
- 4.7g Carbs;
- 0.1g Fiber;
- 19.6g Protein;
- 1.7g Sugars

Fixings:

- 1/2-pound breakfast sausage
- 1/2 cup almond flour
- 1/2 cup Colby cheese, shredded
- 4 tablespoons Romano cheese, freshly grated
- 1 egg
- 1 garlic clove, pressed
- 2 tablespoons fresh chives, minced

Headings

Totally join all trimmings in a mixing bowl; mix until everything is especially combined.

Shape the mix into balls and sort out them on a material lined treat sheet. Heat in the preheated oven at 360 degrees F for around 18 minutes.

Serve warm or cold. Bon appétit!

VEGGIE LOVER

52. MEXICAN INSPIRED STUFFED PEPPERS

Prepared in around: 45 minutes

Servings: 3

These veggie darling stuffed peppers are stacked up with cheddar, eggs, and flavors, then, cooked in the tomato-mustard sauce. You can standard gurgling toll peppers in a salted, percolating water at first.

Per serving:

- 194 Calories;
- 13.9g Fat;
- 3.5g Carbs;
- 0.7g Fiber;
- 13.3g Protein;
- 2.4g Sugars

Fixings:

- 4 bell peppers, halved, seeds removed
- 4 eggs, whisked
- 1 cup Mexican cheese blend
- 1 teaspoon chili powder
- 1 garlic clove, minced
- 1 teaspoon onion powder
- 1 ripe tomato, pureed
- 1 teaspoon mustard powder

Headings

Start by preheating your oven to 370 degrees F. Spritz the base and sides of a baking dish with a cooking oil.

In a mixing bowl, totally unite the eggs, cheddar, stew powder, garlic, and onion powder. Split the filling between the ring peppers.

Mix the tomatoes in with mustard powder and move the blend to the baking holder. Cover with foil and plan for 40 minutes, until the peppers are fragile and the filling is completely warmed. Bon appétit!

53. FRITTATA WITH ASPARAGUS AND HALLOUMI

Prepared in around: 25 minutes

Servings: 4

Halloumi is semi-hard cheddar delivered utilizing a blend of goat's and sheep's milk that is extensively used in Greek cooking. Its significantly flawless flavor goes with eggs and asparagus well for sure.

Per serving:

- 376 Calories;
- 29.1g Fat;
- 4g Carbs;
- 1g Fiber;
- 24.5g Protein;
- 2.5g Sugars

Fixings:

- 1 tablespoon olive oil
- 1/2 red onion, sliced
- 4 ounces asparagus, cut into small chunks
- 1 tomato, chopped
- 5 whole eggs, beaten
- 9 ounces Halloumi cheese, crumbled
- 2 tablespoons green olives, pitted and sliced
- 1 tablespoon fresh parsley, chopped

Headings

Heat the oil in a skillet over medium-high hotness; then, cook the onion and asparagus around 3 minutes, blending continually.

Then, at that point, add the tomato and cook for 2 minutes longer. Move the sautéed vegetables to a baking holder that is gently lubed with cooking oil.

Mix the eggs in with cheddar until generally merged. Pour the mix over the vegetables. Scatter cut olives over the top. Heat in the preheated oven at 350 degrees F for 15 minutes.

Brighten with new parsley and serve immediately. Appreciate!

54. ARRANGED EGGS AND CHEESE IN AVOCADO

Prepared in around: 20 minutes

Servings: 4

Here are journey excellent veggie sweetheart snack! Asiago cheddar adds a staggering faithfulness to these avocado shells like an enchanted that ties everything.

Per serving:

- 300 Calories;
- 24.6g Fat;
- 5.4g Carbs;
- 4.6g Fiber;
- 14.9g Protein;
- 0.5g Sugars

Fixings:

- 1 avocado, pitted and halved
- 3 eggs Sea salt and freshly ground black pepper, to taste
- 1 cup Asiago cheese, grated
- 1/2 teaspoon red pepper flakes
- 1/2 teaspoon dried rosemary
- 1 tablespoon fresh chives, chopped

Headings

Break the eggs into the avocado parts, keeping the yolks immaculate. Sprinkle with salt and dull pepper.

Top with cheddar, red pepper pieces, and rosemary. Arrange the stuffed avocado parts in a baking compartment.

Plan in the preheated oven at 420 degrees F for around 15 minutes. Serve decorated with new chives. Appreciate!

55. TWO-CHEESE ZUCCHINI GRATIN

Prepared in around: 50 minutes

Servings: 5

Accepting you find your gratin watery after the 40 minutes, turn the temperature to 350 degrees F and plan for 10 minutes longer. Permit it to sit something like 20 minutes before cutting and serving.

Per serving:

- 371 Calories;
- 32g Fat;
- 5.2g Carbs;
- 0.3g Fiber;
- 15.7g Protein;
- 2.6g Sugars

Fixings:

- 10 large eggs
- 4 tablespoons yogurt
- 2 zucchinis, sliced
- 1/2 medium-sized leek, sliced Sea salt and ground black pepper, to taste
- 1 teaspoon cayenne pepper
- 1 cup cream cheese
- 3 garlic cloves, minced
- 1 cup Swiss cheese, shredded

Headings

Start by preheating your oven to 360 degrees F. Then, spritz the base and sides of an oven proof skillet with a nonstick cooking shower.

Then, mix the eggs in with yogurt until generally merged.

Get north of 1/2 of the zucchini and leek cuts in the holder. Season with salt, dull pepper, and cayenne pepper. Add cream cheddar and minced garlic.

Add the extra zucchini cuts and leek. Add the egg blend. Top with Swiss cheddar. Heat for 40 minutes, until the top is splendid brown. Bon appétit!

56. ITALIAN ZUPPA DI POMODORO

Prepared in around: 30 minutes

Servings: 3

This Italian-animated soup is stacked with malignant growth counteraction specialist and supplement thick vegetables similarly as various aromatics.

Per serving:

- 137 Calories;
- 10.7g Fat;
- 5.6g Carbs;
- 1.2g Fiber;
- 5.6g Protein;
- 2.4g Sugars

Fixings:

- 4 ounces broccoli
- 2 tablespoons sesame oil
- 1 small-sized onion, chopped
- 2 garlic cloves, minced
- 1 teaspoon cayenne pepper
- Sea salt and ground black pepper, to taste
- 1 cup spinach leaves, torn into pieces
- 1 celery stalk, peeled and chopped
- 2 cups vegetable broth
- 1 cup water
- 1 tomato, pureed
- 1 jalapeno pepper, minced
- 1 tablespoon Italian seasonings

Headings

Beat the broccoli in your food processor until rice-sized pieces are outlined; work in packs; hold.

Then, heat the oil in a pot over medium hotness. Then, sauté the onion and garlic until fragile and fragrant.

Add the broccoli and cook for 2 minutes more. Add the extra trimmings, yet, the spinach.

Bring to a quick air pocket and thereafter, straightaway decrease the hotness to medium-low. By and by, stew the soup around 25 minutes.

Add spinach, switch off the hotness, and cover with the top; let it shrink. Bon appétit!

57. TWO-CHEESE AND KALE BAKE

Prepared in around: 35 minutes

Servings: 4

This veggie darling hotness is pouring out done with cheddar and kale; it's so enhancing and engaging. You can use your treasured kind of cheddar. Appreciate!

Per serving:

- 384 Calories;
- 29.1g Fat;
- 5.9g Carbs;
- 1.5g Fiber;
- 25.1g Protein;
- 1.8g Sugars

Fixings:

- Nonstick cooking spray
- 6 ounces kale, torn into pieces
- 3 eggs, whisked
- 1 cup Cheddar cheese, grated
- 1 cup Romano cheese
- 2 tablespoons sour cream
- 1 garlic clove, minced Sea salt, to taste
- 1/2 teaspoon ground black pepper, or more to taste
- 1/2 teaspoon cayenne pepper

Headings

Start by preheating your oven to 365 degrees F. Spritz the sides and lower part of a baking holder with a nonstick cooking sprinkle.

Mix all trimmings and void the mix into the baking holder.

Plan for 30 to 35 minutes or until it is totally warmed. Bon appétit!

58. GRANDMA'S ZUCCHINI AND SPINACH CHOWDER

Prepared in around: 25 minutes

Servings: 4

Keto plans don't come much less difficult than this more seasoned style, veggie darling chowder. You can change it with your dearest flavors and keto mix ins.

Per serving:

- 85 Calories;
- 5.9g Fat;
- 3.8g Carbs;
- 1.3g Fiber;
- 3.7g Protein;
- 1.2g Sugars

Fixings:

- 1 tablespoon olive oil
- 1 clove garlic, chopped
- 1/2 cup scallions, chopped
- 4 cups water
- 2 zucchinis, sliced
- 1 celery stalk, chopped
- 2 tablespoons vegetable bouillon powder
- 4 ounces baby spinach
- Salt and ground black pepper, to taste
- 1 heaping tablespoon fresh parsley, chopped
- 1 tablespoon butter
- 1 egg, beaten

Headings

In a stockpot, heat the oil over medium-high hotness. As of now, cook the garlic and scallions until sensitive or around 4 minutes.

Add water, zucchini, celery, vegetable bouillon powder; cook for 13 minutes.

Add spinach, salt, dim pepper, parsley, and margarine; cook for a further 5 minutes.

Then, blend in the egg and mix until particularly merged. Scoop into individual dishes and serve warm. Appreciate!

TIDBITS and APPETIZERS

59. LETTUCE WRAPS WITH HAM AND CHEESE

Prepared in around: 10 minutes

Servings: 5

You can use frosty mass lettuce or even spinach and chard in this equation. Set up this direct recipe early and participate in your party unbounded.

Per serving:

- 148 Calories;
- 10.2g Fat;
- 4.2g Carbs;
- 0.8g Fiber;
- 10.7g Protein;
- 2.5g Sugars

Fixings:

- 10 Boston lettuce leaves, washed and rinsed well
- 1 tablespoon lemon juice, freshly squeezed
- 11 tablespoons cream cheese
- 10 thin ham slices
- 1 tomato, chopped.
- 1 red chili pepper, chopped

Headings

Sprinkle lemon juice over the lettuce leaves. Spread cream cheddar over the lettuce leaves. Add a ham cut on each leaf.

Split cut tomatoes between the lettuce leaves. Top with stew peppers and coordinate on a fair serving platter. Bon appétit!

60. RANCH AND BLUE CHEESE DIP

Prepared in around: 10 minutes

Servings: 10

This tart plunging sauce goes immaculately with chicken wings or vegetable sticks. Get your starter right with this quick and basic equation!

Per serving:

- 94 Calories;
- 8.1g Fat;
- 1.3g Carbs;
- 0.1g Fiber;
- 4.1g Protein;
- 0.7g Sugars

Fixings:

- 1/2 cup Greek-style yogurt
- 1 cup blue cheese, crumbled
- 1/2 cup mayonnaise
- 1 tablespoon lime juice Freshly ground black pepper, to taste
- 2 tablespoons ranch seasoning

Headings

In a mixing bowl totally solidify all trimmings until generally joined. Function admirably for chilled with your most cherished keto scoops. Bon appétit!

61. RANCH CHICKEN WINGS

Prepared in around: 55 minutes

Servings: 6

The most remarkable viewpoint, these wings are quite easy to make and flexible to your own taste tendencies. Your guests will be returning for extra.

Per serving:

- 466 Calories;
- 37.2g Fat;
- 1.9g Carbs;
- 0.1g Fiber;
- 28.6g Protein;
- 0.7g Sugars

Fixings:

- 2 pounds chicken wings, pat dry Nonstick cooking spray Sea salt and cayenne pepper, to taste
- Ranch Dressing:
- 1/4 cup sour cream
- 1/4 cup buttermilk
- 1/2 cup mayonnaise
- 1/2 teaspoon lemon juice
- 1 tablespoon fresh parsley, minced
- 1 clove garlic, minced
- 2 tablespoons onion, finely chopped
- 1/4 teaspoon dry mustard Sea salt and ground black pepper, to taste

Headings

Start by preheating your oven to 420 degrees F.

Spritz the chicken wings with a cooking shower. Sprinkle the chicken wings with salt and cayenne pepper. Arrange the chicken wings on a material lined baking dish.

Heat in the preheated oven for 50 minutes or until the wings is splendid and new.

In the interim, make the dressing by mixing all of the above trimmings. Present with warm wings.

62. COLBY CHEESE-STUFFED MEATBALLS

Prepared in around: 25 minutes

Servings: 8

Mozzarella 3D shapes tucked inside meatballs! Serve these meatballs on a bed of new zucchini noodles (zoodles).

Per serving:

- 389 Calories;
- 31.3g Fat;
- 1.6g Carbs;
- 0.5g Fiber;
- 23.8g Protein;
- 0.8g Sugars

Fixings:

- 1/2-pound ground pork
- 1 pound ground turkey
- 1 garlic clove, minced
- 4 tablespoons pork rinds, crushed
- 2 tablespoons shallots, chopped
- 5 ounces mozzarella string cheese, cubed
- 1 ripe tomato, pureed Salt and ground black pepper, to taste

Headings

In a mixing bowl totally unite all trimmings, except for the cheddar. Shape the blend into downsized balls.

Press 1 cheddar 3D shape into the point of convergence of each ball.

Set the meatballs on a material lined baking sheet. Plan in the preheated oven at 350 degrees F for 18 to 25 minutes. Bon appétit!

63. CHEDDAR AND ARTICHOKE DIP

Prepared in around: 25 minutes

Servings: 10

This notable dunk gets together in less than 25 minutes. What's more who can anytime deny this rich goodness?

Per serving:

- 367 Calories;
- 31.7g Fat;
- 5.1g Carbs;
- 2.4g Fiber;
- 16.2g Protein;
- 1.7g Sugars

Fixings:

- 10 ounces canned artichoke hearts, drained and chopped
- 6 ounces cream cheese
- 1/2 cup Greek-style yogurt
- 1/2 cup mayo
- 1/2 cup water
- 2 cloves garlic, minced
- 20 ounces Monterey-Jack cheese, shredded

Headings

Start by preheating your oven to 350 degrees F.

Merge the trimmings as a rule, beside the Monterey-Jack cheddar. Place the blend in a gently lubed baking dish.

Top with the obliterated Monterey-Jack cheddar. Heat in the preheated oven for 17 to 22 minutes or until bubbly. Serve warm.

64. ITALIAN CHEESE CRISPS

Prepared in around: 10 minutes

Servings: 4

Direct and fun, with just 5 minutes prep, these crisps are significantly improved and more grounded than excellent potato chips or some other took care of snack you can find.

Per serving:

- 134 Calories;
- 11.1g Fat;
- 0.4g Carbs;
- 4.9g Protein;

Fixings:

- 1 cup sharp Cheddar cheese, grated
- 1/4 teaspoon ground black pepper
- 1/2 teaspoon cayenne pepper
- 1 teaspoon Italian seasoning

Headings

Start by preheating an oven to 400 degrees F. Line a baking sheet with a material paper.

Mix all of the above trimmings until generally combined.

Then, place tablespoon-sized heaps of the mix onto the coordinated baking sheet.

Get ready at the preheated oven for 8 minutes, until the edges start to brown.

License the cheddar crisps to cool fairly; then, put them in writing towels to exhaust the excess fat. Appreciate!

65. FLAVORED EGGS WITH MUSTARD AND CHIVES

Prepared in around: 20 minutes + chilling time

Servings: 8

These stuffed eggs are obviously appropriate for party dinners and potlucks. A cook's note: Once the eggs are chilled, break them and spot in cool water for 10 minutes; the strips will tumble off significantly easier.

Per serving:

- 149 Calories;
- 11.3g Fat;
- 1.6g Carbs;
- 0.1g Fiber;
- 9.4g Protein;
- 1g Sugars

Fixings:

- 7 eggs
- 2 tablespoons cream cheese
- 1 teaspoon Dijon mustard
- 1 tablespoon mayonnaise
- 1 tablespoon tomato puree, no sugar added
- 1 teaspoon balsamic vinegar Sea salt and freshly ground black pepper, to taste
- 1/4 teaspoon cayenne pepper
- 2 tablespoons chives, chopped

Headings

Place the eggs in a single layer in a pot. Add water to cover the eggs and hotness with the end result of bubbling.

Cover, switch off the hotness, and let the eggs address 15 minutes. Channel the eggs and strip them under crisp running water.

Slice the eggs down the middle longwise; kill the yolks and totally unite them with cream cheddar, mustard, mayo, tomato puree, vinegar, salt, dull, and cayenne pepper.

Then, at that point, split the yolk mix between egg whites. Adorn with new chives and appreciate!

66. MINUSCULE STUFFED PEPPERS

Prepared in around: 15 minutes

Servings: 5

Who says stuffed peppers ought to be held for early afternoon? These more modest than regular fiery eats will enchant your guests!

Per serving:

- 198 Calories;
- 17.2g Fat;
- 3g Carbs;
- 0.9g Fiber;
- 7.8g Protein;
- 1.8g Sugars

Fixings:

- 2 teaspoons olive oil
- 1 teaspoon mustard seeds
- 4 ounces ground turkey
- Salt and ground black pepper, to taste
- 10 mini bell peppers, cut in half lengthwise, stems and seeds removed
- 2 ounces garlic and herb seasoned chevron goat cheese, crumbled

Headings

Heat the oil in a skillet over medium-high hotness. Once hot, cook mustard seeds with ground turkey until the turkey are as of now not pink. Crumble with a fork.

Season with salt and dim pepper.

Lay the pepper parts cut-side-up on a material lined baking sheet. Spoon the meat mix into the point of convergence of each pepper half.

Top each pepper with cheddar. Plan in the preheated oven at 400 degrees F for 10 minutes. Bon appétit!

TREATS

67. ALMOND BUTTER AND CHOCOLATE COOKIES

Prepared in around: 15 minutes + chilling time

Servings: 8

This is no get ready, keto-obliging, and fundamental treat for any occasion! Use coconut oil cooking shower to delicately lube a baking sheet; it will allow you to viably cut and dispose of the squares from the baking sheet.

Per serving:

- 322 Calories;
- 28.9g Fat;
- 3.4g Carbs;
- 0.6g Fiber;
- 13.9g Protein;
- 0.7g Sugars

Fixings:

- 1 stick butter
- 1/2 cup almond butter
- 1/2 cup Monk fruit powder
- 4 cups pork rinds, crushed
- 1 teaspoon vanilla extract
- 1/4 teaspoon ground cinnamon
- 1/2 cup sugar-free chocolate, cut into chunks
- 1/2 cup double cream

Headings

In a dish condense the margarine, almond spread, and Monk normal item powder over medium hotness. By and by, add the crushed pork skins and vanilla. Set the hitter on a treat sheet and let it cool in your refrigerator. In the meantime, in a little dish over medium hotness, melt the chocolate and twofold cream. Add the chocolate layer over the player. Grant it to chill absolutely preceding cutting and serving. Bon appétit!

68. ESSENTIAL ORANGE CHEESECAKE

Prepared in around: 15 minutes + chilling time

Servings: 12

This cheesecake represents a flavor like all that you love about Christmas season yet without an unreasonable number of calories and sugar. Similarly, this treat doesn't anticipate that you should go through hours in the kitchen.

Per serving:

- 150 Calories;
- 15.4g Fat;
- 2.1g Carbs;
- 0.1g Fiber;
- 1.2g Protein;
- 1.9g Sugars

Fixings

Outside:

- 1 tablespoon Swerve
- 1 cup almond flour
- 1 stick spread room temperature
- 1/2 cup unsweetened coconut, destroyed

Filling:

- 1 teaspoon powdered gelatin
- 2 tablespoons Swerve
- 17 ounces mascarpone cream
- 2 tablespoon squeezed orange

Headings

Totally join all of the components for the structure; press the covering mix into a delicately lubed baking dish. Permit it to stay in your refrigerator. Then, mix 1 cup of foaming water and gelatin until all separated. Pour in 1 cup of cold water. Add Swerve, mascarpone cheddar, and crushed orange; blend until smooth and uniform. Pour the filling onto the set up external layer. Appreciate!

69. PEANUT BUTTER AND CHOCOLATE TREAT

Prepared in around: 10 minutes + chilling time

Servings: 10

You can make this sweet early and store it in the cooler until arranged to eat. Participate in the entire flavor without culpability!

Per serving:

- 122 Calories;
- 11.7g Fat;
- 4.9g Carbs;
- 1.4g Fiber;
- 1.5g Protein;
- 1.9g Sugars

Fixings:

- 1 sticks butter, room temperature
- 1/3 cup peanut butter
- 1/3 cup unsweetened cocoa powder
- 1/3 cup Swerve
- 1/2 teaspoon ground cinnamon A pinch of grated nutmeg
- 1/4 cup unsweetened coconut flakes
- 1/4 cup pork rinds, crushed

Headings

Break down the spread and peanut butter until smooth and uniform.

Add the extra trimmings and mix until everything is generally joined.

Line a baking sheet with a silicone baking mat. Void the blend into the baking sheet. Place in your cooler for 1 hour until arranged to serve. Appreciate!

70. COCONUT CRANBERRY BARS

Prepared in around: 1 hour 10 minutes

Servings: 12

One of nature's most amazing gifts to us is a new and sweet natural item. By and by, we will use coconut and cranberries and make these great bars; with their sensitive and smooth surface, you will add a smidgen of summer to your days.

Per serving:

- 107 Calories;
- 11.1g Fat;
- 2.5g Carbs;
- 0.9g Fiber;
- 0.4g Protein;
- 1.4g Sugars

Fixings:

- 1/3 cup cranberries
- 1 ½ cups coconut flakes, unsweetened
- 1/2 cup butter, melted
- 1/2 teaspoon liquid Stevia

Headings

Mix all trimmings in your food processor until generally joined. Press the hitter into a baking sheet.

Refrigerate for an hour. Cut into bars and function admirably for chilled.

71. NUT AND BUTTER CUBES

Prepared in around: 50 minutes

Servings: 10

With its fragile and crunchy surface, these nut 3D squares are a treat sweetheart's dream. You can't get enough of them.

Per serving:

- 218 Calories;
- 21.2g Fat;
- 5.1g Carbs;
- 0.7g Fiber;
- 3.8g Protein;
- 1.3g Sugars

Fixings:

- 1 stick butter
- 1/3 cup coconut oil
- 1 vanilla paste
- 1/4 teaspoon cinnamon powder
- 2 tablespoons Monk fruit powder A pinch of coarse salt
- 1/2 cup peanuts, toasted and coarsely chopped

Headings

Microwave the spread, coconut oil, and vanilla until melted. Add cinnamon powder, Monk regular item powder, and salt.

Put the hacked peanuts into a silicon structure or an ice strong shape plate. Pour the warm spread blend over the peanuts.

Place in your cooler for 40 to 50 minutes. Bon appétit!

72. LEAST COMPLEX BROWNIES EVER

Prepared in around: 1 hour

Servings: 10

To use a microwave, just convey water to a stew. Place the heatproof bowl over the pot with high temp water; guarantee the water doesn't contact the bowl. Place the chocolate in the bowl and blend discontinuously until it is relaxed.

Per serving:

- 205 Calories;
- 19.5g Fat;
- 5.4g Carbs;
- 3.2g Fiber;
- 4.7g Protein;
- 0.4g Sugars

Fixings:

- 1 tablespoon almond flour
- 3 tablespoons coconut flour
- 1/2 teaspoon baking powder
- 1/2 cup cocoa powder, unsweetened
- 4 eggs
- 1/2 cup Swerve
- 1 teaspoon almond extract
- 1 vanilla extract
- 1/2 cup coconut oil
- 4 ounces baking chocolate, unsweetened

Headings

Totally unite the almond flour, coconut flour, cocoa powder, and baking powder.

Mix in the eggs, Swerve, almond and vanilla concentrate; beat with an electric blender on high until everything is generally joined.

In an alternate bowl, disintegrate the coconut oil and chocolate in your microwave. Yet again as of now, add the egg mix and mix.

Logically add the dry trimmings and race until everything is generally combined. Void the hitter into a delicately lubed baking skillet.

Get ready in the preheated grill at 320 degrees F approximately 50 minutes or until a toothpick installed into the focal point of your brownie comes clean and dry. Bon appétit!

73. NO BAKE PARTY CAKE

Prepared in around: 30 minutes

Servings: 6

The ideal party cake, Irish cream cheesecake is a model treat that everyone will appreciate. It makes a basic birthday cake, too.

Per serving:

- 274 Calories;
- 27.5g Fat;
- 5.7g Carbs;
- 1.6g Fiber;
- 3.8g Protein;
- 2.1g Sugars

Fixings:

- 1/4 cup almond flour
- 1/4 cup coconut flour
- 2 tablespoons cocoa powder
- 1 ½ tablespoons Swerve
- 1 tablespoon almond butter
- 2 tablespoons coconut oil A pinch of salt
- A pinch of cinnamon powder
- 7 ounces mascarpone cheese
- 2 tablespoons coconut oil
- 2 tablespoons cocoa powder
- 1/4 cup tablespoons Swerve
- 1/3 cup double cream
- 2 tablespoons Irish whiskey
- 1 teaspoon vanilla extract
- 1/2 cup double cream
- 1 teaspoon grass-fed gelatin

Headings

In a little bowl totally combine the almond flour, coconut flour, cocoa, and Swerve.

Add almond spread, coconut oil, salt, and cinnamon powder; press the outside into a baking compartment.

To make the filling, condense mascarpone cheddar and coconut oil in a microwave for 40 seconds.

Add cocoa, Swerve, 1/3 cup of cream, Irish whiskey, and vanilla; beat with an electric blender until smooth and uniform.

Then, whip 1/2 cup of twofold cream until it has increased in volume.

In a little mixing bowl, get gelatin together with 1 tablespoon of cold water; rush until separated. By and by, add 1 tablespoon of high temp water and blend until particularly solidified.

Steadily and gradually, add separated gelatin to the whipped cream; mix until strong. By and by, overlay the coordinated whipped cream into the cream cheddar blend.

Spread the filling over the external layer and function admirably for chilled. Appreciate!

74. VANILLA MUG CAKE

Prepared in around: 10 minutes

Servings: 2

All of the trimmings are consolidated as one, and a short time later your cakes cook in the microwave for around 1 second. In like manner, there are limitless combinations of flavors; you can add normal items, cocoa, chocolate, and different flavors. Basic!

Per serving:

- 143 Calories;
- 10.7g Fat;
- 5.7g Carbs;
- 2.6g Fiber;
- 5.7g Protein;
- 2.8g Sugars

Fixings:

- 3 tablespoons psyllium husk flour
- 2 tablespoons ground flax seed
- 4 tablespoons almond flour
- 5 tablespoons Monk fruit powder A pinch of salt A pinch of grated nutmeg
- 1 teaspoon baking soda
- 5 tablespoons full-fat milk
- 1 teaspoon vanilla paste

Headings

Totally solidify all of the above trimmings in delicately lubed mugs. Then, microwave your cakes for 1 second. Bon appétit!

THANK YOU

Made in the USA
Middletown, DE
25 April 2022

64735724R00066